Palgrave Studies in Literary Anthropology

Series Editors
Deborah Reed-Danahay
Department of Anthropology
The State University of New York at Buffalo
Buffalo, NY, USA

Helena Wulff
Department of Social Anthropology
Stockholm University
Stockholm, Sweden

This series explores new ethnographic objects and emerging genres of writing at the intersection of literary and anthropological studies. Books in this series are grounded in ethnographic perspectives and the broader cross-cultural lens that anthropology brings to the study of reading and writing. The series explores the ethnography of fiction, ethnographic fiction, narrative ethnography, creative nonfiction, memoir, autoethnography, and the connections between travel literature and ethnographic writing.

Robert Desjarlais • Sabina M. Perrino
Joshua O. Reno • Nicholas Bartlett
Aurora Donzelli • Margaux Fitoussi
Alexa Hagerty • Rafadi Hakim
Parthiban Muniandy • Emily Ng

Dispatches from Home and the Field during the COVID-19 Pandemic

palgrave
macmillan

Robert Desjarlais
Department of Anthropology
Sarah Lawrence College
Bronxville, NY, USA

Sabina M. Perrino
Department of Anthropology
Binghamton University
Binghamton, NY, USA

Joshua O. Reno
Department of Anthropology
Binghamton University
Binghamton, NY, USA

Nicholas Bartlett
Asian and Middle Eastern Cultures
Barnard College, Columbia University
New York, NY, USA

Aurora Donzelli
Linguistic Anthropology
Sarah Lawrence College and the
University of Bologna
Bronxville, NY, USA

Margaux Fitoussi
Anthropology
Columbia University
New York City, NY, USA

Alexa Hagerty
University of Cambridge
Cambridge, UK

Rafadi Hakim
University of Chicago
Chicago, IL, USA

Parthiban Muniandy
Department of Sociology
Sarah Lawrence College
Bronxville, NY, USA

Emily Ng
Amsterdam School for Cultural
Analysis
University of Amsterdam
Amsterdam, The Netherlands

Palgrave Studies in Literary Anthropology
ISBN 978-3-031-19192-3 ISBN 978-3-031-19193-0 (eBook)
https://doi.org/10.1007/978-3-031-19193-0

This Palgrave Macmillan imprint is published by the registered company Springer Nature Switzerland AG.
The registered company address is: Gewerbestrasse 11, 6330 Cham, Switzerland

The face of London was—now indeed strangely altered: I mean the whole mass of buildings, city, liberties, suburbs, Westminster, Southwark, and altogether; for as to the particular part called the city, or within the walls, that was not yet much infected. But in the whole the face of things, I say, was much altered; sorrow and sadness sat upon every face; and though some parts were not yet overwhelmed, yet all looked deeply concerned; and, as we saw it apparently coming on, so everyone looked on himself and his family as in the utmost danger.

Daniel Defoe,
A Journal of the Plague Year, 1722

As you can see, the sun is high, the heat intense, and the silence unbroken save by the cicadas in the olive trees. For the moment, it would be the height of folly to quit this spot. Here the air is cool and the prospect fair, and here, observe, are dice and chess. Take, then, your pleasure as you may be severally minded; but, if you take my advice, you will find pastime for the hot hours before us, not in play…but in telling stories, in which the invention of one may afford solace to all the company of his hearers".....The queen's proposal being approved by all, ladies and gentlemen alike, she added: "So please you, then, I ordain, that, for this first day, we should be free to speak on whatever matter we please." She then addressed Panfilo, who was seated to her right, bidding him with a gracious air to lead off with one of his stories. And prompt at the word of command, Panfilo, while all listened intently, thus began.

Giovanni Boccaccio,
The Decameron, 1353

Preface

Writing Viral

The book that you hold in your hands entails a multi-voiced compendium of writing on life during the COVID-19 pandemic, within the strands of first-person, reflective writings authored by ten scholars who work primarily within the fields of anthropology and sociology. The first of our writings began in the Spring of 2020, during those intense and heady initial weeks of the pandemic, as pressing concerns about the coronavirus took form throughout the world. The first series of exchanges occurred over email and Zoom meetings between editors Robert Desjarlais, Sabina M. Perrino, and Joshua O. Reno. This tentative, exploratory conversation soon grew into a sustained dialogue with seven other scholars across the globe, namely Nicholas Bartlett, Aurora Donzelli, Margaux Fitoussi, Alexa Hagerty, Rafadi Hakim, Parthiban Muniandy, and Emily Ng. Month by month, we asked ourselves to write on various formations of the pandemic from our respective vantage points, as we tried, alone and in relation to others, to make sense of and live with the many challenges and possibilities for life during these times.

The short essays, or entries, featuring this book have been spun from diverse situations, contexts, and locations from the United States, be it Oakland, California, Illinois, and upstate, urban, and suburban New York, to dispersedly still, Denmark, England, Italy, France, the Netherlands, and Tunisia, along with the considerations of present-day life in places like China, Malaysia, and Indonesia. Each entry proceeds within a spatiotemporal flow, starting in March 2020, with the first alerts and cases of viral

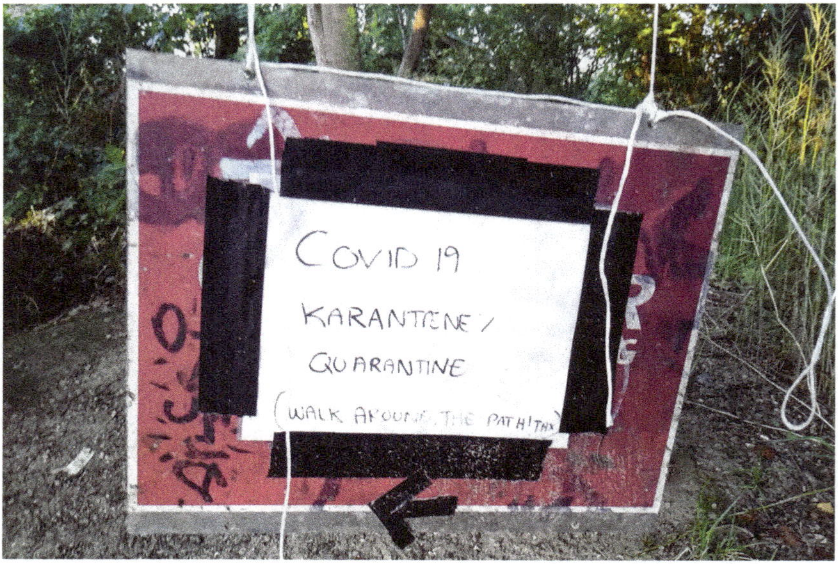

Fig. 1 Quarantine sign, Christiania, Copenhagen, June 2020. (Photo by R. Desjarlais)

infection in various parts of the world, and then moving on to various currents of caution, concern, infection, despair, hope, and connection that have unfolded since those early days. The writings then move into 2021, with events and moods associated with the global distribution of potentially effective vaccines and the promise and hope these immunizations bring. The written record of these multiform reflections involves traces of a series of lives, as the authors of those lives tried to make do, and write, in trying times (Fig. 1).

This collaborative effort has led to something distinct. Rather than an edited volume with dedicated chapters, the current work derives from our process of writing together as a collective for over a year. The format is fitting for the evolving and precarious conditions created by the pandemic. Instead of being asked to devise distinct and comprehensive scholarly chapters, rich in precise expertise and learned reasoning, the contributors to this volume have crafted a number of entries, each brief and compact, with reflections that allow each author' perspectives and stories to emerge, in tandem with the pandemic itself. In this way, our book has a distinctive, emerging multivocality which is not interrupted by the more common division of dedicated, single-authored chapters. This approach thus creates a dynamic flow to the writing throughout, such that the sections of the book are not framed or divided based on abstract themes but, rather, are punctuated by global events and the vicissitudes of pandemic life, including initial reactions to successive "waves" of infection, societies closing down and then opening again (only to shut down again, in ever-shifting circumstances), with the promise of vaccinations emergent on the horizon.

One of the main questions this book asks is: What does it mean to live and write amid an unfolding and unstoppable global health and economic crisis? As we have been writing, people around the world have been socially distanced and confined indoors, and many are writing as well. This is true in terms of a greater reliance on emails, texts, posts, and other digital tools as substitutes for interpersonal interactions, but also is reflected by the explosive growth in personal journals ("From first-time diarists to lifelong notebook enthusiasts, people around the world are jotting down their thoughts in the pandemic"[1]) in newly begun books and memoirs ("Pandemic prose: COVID-19 sparks literary effort"[2]) or, on the more practical side, in the last will and testaments that more people are writing in light of ever-present, everyday death. Across the globe, people are arguably writing more now and with more urgency, be it to communicate with others, leave a clear record behind, get some work done, or to reflect creatively on the actualities of the pandemic.

Dispatches from Home and the Field during the COVID-19 Pandemic begins with the sobering thought that during a pandemic—and, more generally, in all times—writing is both remedy and poison. In keeping with Jacques Derrida's translation of Plato's *pharmakon*, there is something about writing that "doesn't come from around here. It comes from afar, it is external or alien: to the living, which is the right-here of the inside, to the *logos* as the *zöon* it claims to assist or relieve."[3] Writing is virus-like, in that it is not so much a danger to one's body as it is indifferent to whether we live or die and will use up our corporeal resources for its own ends as needed. Writing, in this sense, may be intersubjective but it is also subsubjective, potentially dissolving ourselves in alien alphabetic acids even as we attempt to lay our "real" selves bare. Perhaps this explains why, at the same time as there has been a veritable explosion in writing, levels of anxiety, depression, and mental illness have also been growing in concert (as the US Center of Disease Control reports).[4] In this regard, we should not be so quick to decide whether writing is best classified here as symptom, cure, or cause.

Soon after the beginning of the COVID-19 pandemic, we shared our writing with one another, in the hopes that we might go "beyond the lonely anthropologist" evident in so much ethnographic writing.[5] At first, there were five authors, then eight, and then ten, with each person drawing from their acumen in the fields of, variably, linguistic, medical, and sociocultural anthropology, literature, philosophy, sociology, the arts, and photography. The connections involved were often circumstances of accident and network; along with diasporic intimacies that emerged as if seemingly by chance, with friendships created and sustained through trying times. The dynamics of our collective writing thus mirrored emerging forms of (non)sociality triggered by the pandemic. New friendships as well as disconnections were created through viral fractures and relations. We made new friends, but also lost others. Emergent from these correspondences is a rhizomatic network of friends and colleagues who share a sympathy toward writing about perceptions and experiences in tangible, intensive, less recognizably "scholarly" ways. We were virtual comrades, in Jodi Dean's use of the term, somehow "on the same side" if never under the same roof.[6] Looking back at our collaboration, our conviction now is that, if writing—ethnographic or otherwise—has always presented the troubling possibilities of reflecting on and in life, then pandemic times create an opportunity to think with and through writing in new ways. In short, how does the COVID-19 pandemic change or redirect our attention to the dissolution of the fictitious singular "self," long held suspect, if directed toward the implosion of affective and communicative relations that emerge, unexpectedly, irresistibly, in challenging times of radical and global change? How might then authors speak to the sundry challenges, concerns, and wayward perceptions that arise through the tremulous course of a pandemic of such proportions?

Dispatches is the product of a novel collaborative endeavor to delve into forms of writing in "real time" during emergent moments of a global crisis. From the start, we thought of our writings as *dispatches* of various sorts—informal, personal communiqués, written from a plurality of locations and contexts, through words that carried a sense of immediacy, of direct relevance to the lives and deaths under consideration. There is a distinct literary form to a dispatch, which is unlike the entries of a journal, or an ethnographer's fieldnotes, which are chiefly written by and for the ethnographer herself, as notes only. A dispatch is also unlike any of the news updates rifling through the media these days (as with the constantly updated, "Here's what you need to know" posts on the "live" website of *The New York Times*). A dispatch implies something "dispatched" quickly, something "sent off" or "sent out"—or something "dismissed," or "disposed of properly,"—done away with, even. There's an air of a message and a messenger in any written dispatch, words are penned and sent off, dispatched, intended to be read by others. The text of a dispatch is like a flash, a flare, a blast, an SOS, or a message in a bottle, drifting upon a lonely ocean expanse, possibly but not necessarily reaching a reader, continents away. A dispatch is usually geared toward a public, toward a readership that is direct and immediate, or potential, abstract, or imagined only. The dispatch can involve a form of emergency-driven first-person writing, which turns the self and its grounds into an object of observation, and, often, is addressed to a generic, unknown, potential reader/addressee. There is a sense of urgency and now-time quality to a dispatch. The dispatch tends to evoke a powerful mixture of first-person testimony awareness (and alienation, at times), as in writing on the edge of disaster, in a time of catastrophe, or in scenes of conflict. And unlike the crucially important reporting of journalists, there is an air of anthropological reflectiveness—and anxious rumination, at times—with our dispatches. Accordingly, we have written within the urgent temporalities and intensive language of what might be called dispatch ethnography.[7]

Through the course of 2020, and then on into 2021 and, briefly, 2022, contributors have shared and circulated their candid reflections on the global COVID-19 pandemic as it has been unfolding through the lenses of their everyday lives. The brief and singular essays preserve the sense of urgency, uncertainty, and open-endedness of diverse subjective experiences and intersubjective engagements. The *viral* is both subject and method here; along with relating to the processes and effects of the COVID-19 virus, the writing, through time, has proceeded in decidedly viral forms: one person's dispatch led to another's reflection, the potent glean of an image spawned further images, within a discourse-contagion of thought, affect, image. In time, the *variant* became a motif; just as the COVID-19 virus has been taking on new viral forms, issuing novel "variants of concern" in the world (Alpha, Delta, Omicron B1 and B2, etc.), and with life more generally shifting into new emergent forms of relation and becoming, illness, and possible well-being—like a kaleidoscope that keeps shifting into new arrangements of optical form with each new rotation of a multi-reflector device—so each new series of dispatches appeared like novel variants of thought and experience, adding to what came before, shifting the terms of perception.

Above all, we have tried to pay attention to the *intensities* of everyday life, and to the affects that course through our days and nights and those of others: grief, sadness, worry, concern, anxiety, fear, loneliness, isolation, hope, joy, anticipation, senses of uncertainty, and meditations on death—the "ordinary affects" of extraordinary times, as it were.[8] The intensities involved are at once kinetic (the rapid speed of events, exponential contagion, the acceleration of "number streams," keeping tracking of viral rates and new variants, along with the slowing down of daily practices and interactions), temporal (speeds and slownesses, variable recurrence, the déjà-vu-like, *déjà-covid* quality of many coronavirus-governance patterns, the eternal return of restriction), acoustic/sonic (the sounds and silences of pandemic life), corporeal (symptom, sensation, contact, isolation), tactile (proximity, touch, and the absence of touch), material (masks, jabs, intangible but highly dangerous viruses, the lonely companionship of food, coffee, games, books, podcasts, Netflix), and relational (yearning for moments among others while fearful of such proximities and potential intimacies). Such first-person and interpersonal reflections touch on a plurality of themes brought on by the pandemic, forces, and dynamics of pressing concern to many, such as contagion, safety, health inequalities, societal injustices, loss and separation, displacement, phantasmal imaginings and possibilities, the uncertain arts of calculating risk and protection, limits on movement and travel, and the biopolitical operations of sovereign powers. Different, intersecting scales of life, pathology, and governmentality are implied: the granular, micrologic scale of the writing proceeds within a backdrop of events at a more macro-level—from "viral spread" and the nation-wide, government-enforced shutdowns and travel bans to health disparities and the depletion of medical resources in certain communities, and the deaths of many. With this, certain structures of attention recur; major events tend to lie in the background, while the intensity and extensity of minor details are foregrounded. (Auto)ethnography here is not just a style of writing, but a crystalized form of lived experience.

These are fragile texts. They are written in situations of existential and social precarity, of vulnerability, within swirls of pandemic anxiety and fatigue, in situations where the right next steps were uncertain and the future viability of oneself and loved ones was thrown into question. With this anxious poetics, weariness and exhaustion sometimes underpin the mood of the writing. We wrote, in fact, until we grew tired of writing, tired of thinking and writing intensively about the pandemic, the world of this text ends with a sigh. An air of vulnerability and exposure might therefore transfer over into any receptions of this volume. When it came to editing and revising the dispatches with an eye toward publication, we tried to maintain the fragility of the texts, and refrained from polishing them too much or fashioning them into perfected expert treatises. There is an immediacy here, a rawness to which, we believe, many persons who have lived through a pandemic can relate.

Because each section of the book coalesces around specific times, spaces, and events in the growth and spread of the COVID-19 pandemic, we also offer additional, conditional, short prefaces to each part. We trust that these will help orient the reader as they find their way through our dispatches. In some cases, readers might use this as a means to read the book out of order or to avoid some topics that they are not ready to revisit. No less than writing, reading too can be poison and cure.

Viral times call for viral writing. The many life moments, experiences, and stories that give life to this multivocal book are unique to this historical moment. Pandemics of such proportions do not happen often, but they do leave indelible marks in humans' lives and souls as other natural disasters and traumatic events do. The embodied writings from the contemporary moment will likely be read and told in future times. They will be recounted to children and grandchildren. Perhaps they will become part of new pandemic feelings of dread, fear, isolation, uncertainty, immobility, and hope and creative living in other future, trying times.

Bronxville, NY, USA — Robert Desjarlais
Binghamton, NY, USA — Sabina M. Perrino
Binghamton, NY, USA — Joshua O. Reno

Notes

1. https://www.vox.com/the-goods/21542132/journaling-bullet-journal-coronavirus-pandemic (last accessed, December 30, 2020). See also The Pandemic Journaling Project, a joint initiative of Connecticut University and Brown University; Benedict Carey. 2021. "*'Right Now Feels So Long and Without Any End in Sight,'*" *The New York Times* February 15, 2021.
2. https://www.twincities.com/2020/09/14/pandemic-prose-covid-19-unleashes-literary-outpouring/ (last accessed, December 30, 2020).
3. Derrida (1981: 104).
4. https://www.cdc.gov/mmwr/volumes/69/wr/mm6932a1.htm (last accessed, December 30, 2020).
5. In Alma Gottlieb's (1995) terms.
6. Dean (2019).
7. Michael Herr's *Dispatches* (1977) comes to mind as an exemplar in dispatch. These observations on the literary form and qualities of dispatches draw in particular from the ideas of Aurora Donzelli on the matter, which she generously developed and shared with the authors of this preface.
8. On "ordinary affects," see Stewart (2008).

Contents

About the Authors

Nicholas Bartlett is Assistant Professor in the Department of Asian and Middle Eastern Cultures at Barnard College, Columbia University. He is the author of *Recovering Histories: Life and Labor after Heroin in Reform-era China* (2020). His current research explores the introduction of group relations conferences, a tradition promoting the study of authority and group unconscious processes, to China.

Robert Desjarlais is Professor of Anthropology at Sarah Lawrence College. He is the author of several books, including *Shelter Blues: Sanity and Selfhood among the Homeless*(1997), *Subject to Death: Life and Loss in a Buddhist World* (2016), *The Blind Man: A Phantasmography* (2019), and, co-authored with Khalil Habrih, *Traces of Violence: Writings on the Disaster in Paris, France* (2022). His research interests include the peoples and cultures of the Nepal Himalayas, Tibetan Buddhism, French colonialism, histories of violence, the politics of life and death, and ethnographic writing.

Aurora Donzelli is Associate Professor of Linguistic Anthropology at Sarah Lawrence College and the University of Bologna. Her first monograph—*Methods of Desire* (2019)—examines how neoliberal ideologies are transforming modes of action and ways of speaking among the Toraja highlanders of Indonesia. Her second monograph—*One or Two Words* (2020)—analyzes emerging forms of cosmopolitan indigeneity and novel ways of using language to imagine the nation-state in the Indonesian peripheries. Her new research project among back-to-the-land activists in Italy explores neo-rurality as a response to the post-WWII standardization of both agricultural labor and linguistic interaction. She is the recipient of grants from the NSF, the Wenner-Gren Foundation, and the Portuguese Foundation for Science and Technology.

Margaux Fitoussi is a PhD candidate of Anthropology at Columbia University. She lives between Tunis and New York, and her research interests include the politics of names and naming, personhood, and histories of violence in the Mediterranean. Her films have screened at Film Society of Lincoln Center in New York, Musée d'art et d'histoire du Judaïsme in Paris, Cultural Pinakotheke in Rio de Janeiro and São Paulo, and SAVVY Contemporary in Berlin, among others. Her translations include two volumes of Tunisian Ottoman History and a survey of early Algerian and Tunisian cinema.

Alexa Hagerty is an anthropologist and STS scholar. Her research uses participatory, ethnographic, and arts-based methods to investigate the meeting of bodies and technology in forensics, biometric surveillance, and AI resistance movements. She is an associate fellow at the University of Cambridge, and a senior researcher in JUST AI network of the London School of Economics. In addition to academic publications, she has written for *Wired, Los Angeles Review of Books,* and *Palais de Tokyo.* Her book *Still Life with Bones: Genocide, Forensics, and What Remains* is forthcoming.

Rafadi Hakim is a PhD candidate of Anthropology at the University of Chicago. His research examines how the exchange of words, money, and other value-laden signs undergirds democracy's ethical problems and paradoxes in Kupang, eastern Indonesia.

Parthiban Muniandy is a faculty member of Sociology at Sarah Lawrence College. He is the author of *Ghost Lives of the Pendatang: Informality and Cosmopolitan Contaminations in Urban Malaysia (2021)* and *Politics of the Temporary: An Ethnography of Migrant Life in Urban Malaysia (2015).* His main research interests are in urban life of displaced, undocumented, and hidden communities in Southeast Asia, where he has carried out ethnographic fieldwork since 2011.

Emily Ng is postdoctoral researcher at the Amsterdam School for Cultural Analysis, University of Amsterdam. She is the author of *A Time of Lost Gods: Mediumship, Madness, and the Ghost after Mao* (2020). With regional attention to China, her research interests include madness and mental illness, subjectivity, cosmopolitics, and how historical worlds and wounds reverberate across geographies and generations.

Sabina M. Perrino is Associate Professor of Anthropology and Linguistics at Binghamton University. She is the author of *Narrating Migration: Intimacies of Exclusion in Northern Italy* (2020), *Research Methods in Linguistic Anthropology* (with Sonya Pritzker; 2022), and *Storytelling in the Digital World* (with Anna De Fina; 2019). She has numerous publications on a wide range of linguistic anthropological topics including racialized language in discursive practices; offline and online narratives; intimacy in interaction; language and migration; language revitalization; transnationalism; language use in ethnomedical encounters (Senegal) and in political discourse (Northern Italy); and research methods in linguistic anthropology.

Joshua O. Reno is Professor in the Department of Anthropology at Binghamton University. He is the author of *Waste Away: Working and Living with a North American Landfill* (2016), *Military Waste: The Unexpected Consequences of Permanent War Readiness* (2019), and with Britt Halvorson, *Imagining the Heartland: White Supremacy and the American Midwest* (2022). He is a socio-cultural anthropologist, and his research interests mostly concern various forms of waste—municipal, mammalian, and militaristic—and their impact on lives, economies, and social movements in the US. He has also done research and written in the fields of critical disability studies, bio-semiotics, and critical race theory.

List of Figures

CHAPTER 1

Part I: The First Wave

Dear _____,
We are writing to see if you might be interested in joining a collaborative writing project with a brief book in mind, tentatively titled "Dispatches-19." The idea is for those involved to write several relatively brief texts that speak to various dimensions and situations related to the COVID-19 pandemic, particularly with attention to the everyday and affective qualities of life in these tumultuous times. These various reflections will be integrated into a larger text, set within various themes and subjects....
April 2020

On the Periphery

I write from a periphery. One of several, in fact. To be more precise, and without finding any security in such precision, I write from a studio apartment in a building set along a side street in Vesterbro, one of the outlying neighborhoods of Copenhagen, Denmark. Beyond the city center, this particular area rests on the edge of the former meatpacking district, since transformed into an open-air arcade of shops and restaurants. The doors of most of these establishments are closed just now. It's unclear when they will open again.

I write peripherally, in a time of uncertainty and anxiety and ever-shifting viral Reproduction Rates, RO 2.5, 1.07, 1.33. There is a virus circulating the world, COVID-19. It has made its spectral way across the globe and is now lighting upon most corners of the world. While news of the Corona outbreak is on everyone's mind, it's terrifically unclear where

R. Desjarlais et al., *Dispatches from Home and the Field during the COVID-19 Pandemic*, Palgrave Studies in Literary Anthropology,
https://doi.org/10.1007/978-3-031-19193-0_1

the pathogens might be at any given moment, whether or not they are in the air that one passes, or breathes in, or if it's clinging to the doorknobs and elevator buttons that mark a trail back home.

Many people wonder if they've already had the virus. There was the flu-like ailment and lingering cough they had back in January, or the sore throat in February, which went away as mysteriously as it arrived. Or that delirium fever that one night, gone by morning. Most continue to worry that they might fall ill with the infection, with death as a possible outcome. It's scary.

I write from certain telling peripheries of space and time. I dwell on the margins of family, friendship, institutional power, within circuits of life and death. I am far from the action. My existence so far hovers well beyond the so-called front lines or any virulent "hot spots" in the world. I have not been near a hospital or health clinic, or any testing centers. I've heard no ambulance sirens sounding desperately through the streets. I've seen no dead bodies piling up, or kept in temporary storage facilities (though I've heard of the mass graves). I'm not sure even where I should go if I were suddenly to fall ill with a fever and sore throat, or lose my sense of taste and smell. Still, it's as if it's around me now, unseen, lingering in the streets below.

The virus is sneaky. Largely invisible and unpredictable, immeasurable, it sneaks up on people, hits them hard. Levels them. There's no respite for some. Others say they experience no symptoms at all. There's quite a range, which adds to the perplexity.

No one knows what the long-term consequences of the infection will be for those who survive it. No one knows for sure if, once you've had it, and supposedly have the resultant antibodies in your blood, you are then forever immune from further infections. But some of those who have recovered from the illness now find comfort in the likelihood that they have immunity, and they go about their days in ways more at ease than others.

No one knows what will happen, or what things will be like in a month or year from now. No one knows whether or not the virus will return with a vengeance in the fall, or next year, or the next. Anyone who tells you anything for sure is a fool.

They are now predicting "wavelets" of viral infections this summer, affecting urban centers like waves ascending onto a shoreline and flowing into the surrounding marshlands.

I arrived in Copenhagen at the start of March 2020. There was distant news then of outbreaks in Seattle, and in the New York City area, along with the intense fight to stop the spread of the virus in China, Hong Kong, and South Korea. But in Europe and North America, it was nothing like it is now. Within days Italy caught on fire, and then Spain, and soon after—with the country's leaders and health experts fearing the worse—the schools and universities in Denmark closed down. Within days, shops, restaurants, and cafes had shut their doors as well. Now, when I bike through central Copenhagen I pass through a ghost shell of the city, and I try to imagine what life was like here before the shutdown, or how it might be like once again (Fig. 1.1).

The building from which I write provides lodging for "ex-pats," namely women and men from elsewhere who have come to Denmark to work or study. Most are here for just a few months or so. Some have young children with them. The structure's hallways and stairwells are vacant most of the time. I had come here from New York, where I most often reside. Each night I read the news from that city and state and try to comprehend

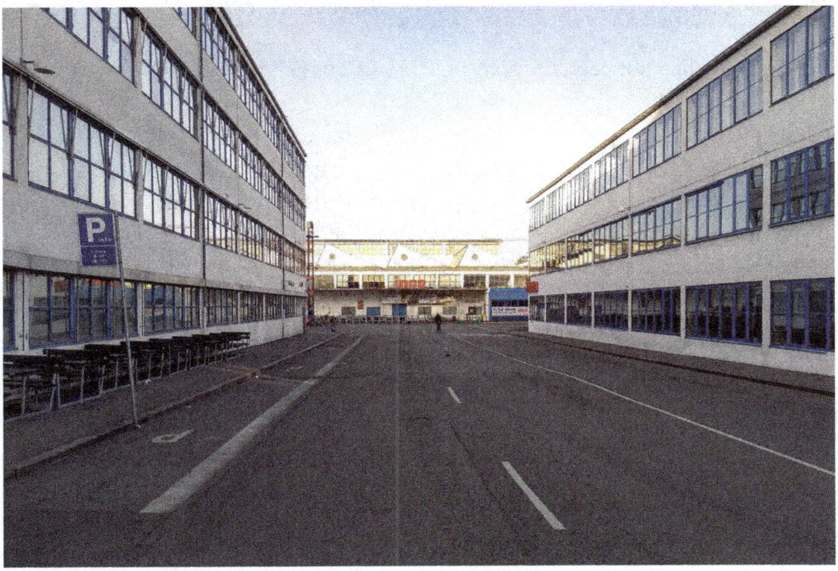

Fig. 1.1 Empty spaces and closed restaurants, Meatpacking area, Copenhagen, April 2020. (Photo by R. Desjarlais)

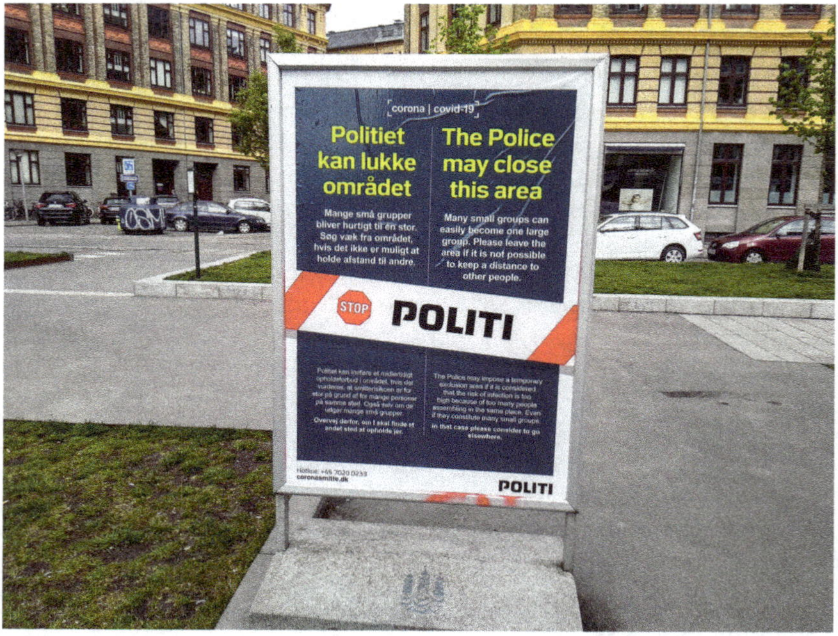
corona | covid-19
Politiet kan lukke området
The Police may close this area
Mange små grupper bliver hurtigt til én stor. Søg væk fra området, hvis det ikke er muligt at holde afstand til andre.
Many small groups can easily become one large group. Please leave the area if it is not possible to keep a distance to other people.
STOP
POLITI
POLITI

Fig. 1.2 Police notice, Copenhagen, April 2020. (Photo by R. Desjarlais)

what it's like to be there now. The high rates of infection have plateaued, but there's still that massive plateau. It appears that most people are staying at home, concerned about going outside. Most wear masks there, now, or so I gather, from images seen online.

All that is far away from here. Others have it much worse, compared to many of us now in Denmark. We're able to go outside when we want to. Few people were masks. It's like the apocalypse has happened and all the people are still around. That doubleness is an odd reality to take in (Fig. 1.2).

Robert Desjarlais

Screen Memories

Early February, 2020. Oakland.

I am driving somewhere. The radio plays an interview with organizers of the Chinese New Year parade in San Francisco, who decided not to cancel the event, unlike those in some other cities, upon hearing news of an unnamed virus spreading in Wuhan. One organizer speaks to how they would provide sanitation precautions—as they *always* have year after year, he notes with subtle emphasis... I picture the organizer on the phone, taking care to keep the irritation on his face from translating into audio traces. Alas, I project. Back on air, a long-time festival goer—a woman, perhaps middle-aged—responds to the reporter, saying that no, she would not be wearing a mask to the event, but notes that those who are concerned can feel free to do so. There was, she seemed to imply, no intrinsic relationship between the effects of the virus on those in Wuhan and Chinese Americans living in San Francisco. Was I projecting again? Was she? Either way, I smile to myself in the car, to what I read as a small moment of refusal—refusal to epidermalize the virus, to blur the principles of Frazerian magic: sympathy and contagion, likeness and nearness.

With all the troubles and contortions of recollection in hindsight, and all those of stumbling along to articulate something not quite articulable in the fog of a still-unfolding moment, I am writing this in August as I try to recall my initial encounters with virus-related matters. It was "just" six months ago, before the concept of a lockdown was fathomable in places like the Bay Area. Before most in the US and in Europe imagined the virus as a creature that could indeed pass through racialized and nationalized borders—so long as one stayed away from Chinatown, many such conversations at the time seemed to hint, one would remain safe, held by whitewashed imaginaries of the nation. But the Chinese—the Sick Man of Asia, as one Wall Street Journal article reminded us with little irony in those days before news of COVID-19's global travels—should perhaps indeed, wear a mask. As images and reports of quarantine in Wuhan saturated US media, conventional accusations of an oriental despotism intensified. Glibness. Righteous disbelief. "*Quarantine*?? You see? China."

Mid-February, 2020. Amsterdam.

I am walking down the hallway at the university. I catch a snippet of conversation as I pause at the printer. "But Italy..." the woman shakes her head. They speak in English. It was an international cluster of academics, some Dutch, some not. The group shares a moment of quiet. News of numbers large enough to scare from within Europe had just begun to solidify. "But..." there was more than one but to be had... "But in some ways, it's not surprising, knowing the way Italy is..." Heads shake, heads nod. Sad, indeed, but... but... with *the way Italy is*... A month later, the

Dutch state would lead a contingent opposing the EU proposal for a "coronabond," which would drive down costs of borrowing for countries most intensely affected by the virus. Facing the arrival of what some had started to call the great equalizer, "the request for solidarity," as one Guardian piece put it, "was swiftly rejected."

Early March, 2020. Amsterdam.

I am sitting on a bench with a group of scholars from Italy. A couple of them note the signs that have been cropping up across the city. "Don't shake hands," one laughs. I show them a photo I had just taken at a bank of one such sign. It was the first time such images began appearing in public spaces in Amsterdam. The numbers in parts of Italy were shooting up. Although two provinces in the north were already shut down, no one there happened to be from those regions. Even as the virus was starting to creep into the homeland, a sense of spatial containability still seemed to squelch the sense of viral mobility, not to mention the still-strong racial-national imaginary of a predominantly Chinese virus. Nonetheless, there was clearly uncertainty in the air. Perceptions were shifting. Many were trying to regain their ground.

"Who are they to say whether we can shake hands?" The notion of a top-down, bureaucratic prohibition of handshakes for a seemingly distant virus brought a small wave of amusement that Amsterdam afternoon—quite Northern, it was implied, and the Dutch were often said to pride themselves in pragmatic planning. I find myself caught, between my own amusement at the new changes and a sense that things in Europe, the US, and wherever else may soon indeed get a lot worse, fast—just as they had in China. Who would still stomach such a laugh then, I think to myself. Then again, the laughter came from those who seemed, at that moment, much closer to the possibility of soon being affected by the contagion than I, as someone based in the US and working in the Netherlands—both relatively untouched by the virus at the time. I would continue to laugh about such signs now and then. But I would also start to stop shaking hands. And they would too.

Late March, 2020. Oakland.

The phrases repeat. Understandably. "This is surreal." "I can't believe this is actually happening." "Nothing is going to be the same after this." *Nothing is going to be the same.* More than other phrases and exclamations, this one stirred something every time it came up—first a reactionary sensation of the need to contradict, followed by the peculiar sensation of an object moving around in my head with no place to go—an awkward long-legged thing that doesn't quite walk and doesn't quite roll. What exactly did everyone think was not going to be the same? And after *what*, exactly? Of course, many answers were given: the economy, education, politics, life as such… and I was not entirely outside of the structures of feeling signaled by such phrases. But to hold that nothing would be the same after a given moment would suggest that there had been some sense of similitude across the moments that came before, and that the future would have otherwise been mapped in the shape of this self-sameness.

Yet again, who am I, who is anyone, to distinguish the not-same from the sensation of not-same by those who live it? "Everything was forever, until it was no more," as Alexei Yurchak described of the beginning of the end of the Soviet Union.[1] The long-legged creature is back, moving listlessly in my head. Stretch—thud. Stretch—thud.

Wade Davis recently wrote a controversial piece on the unraveling of America—that the effects of and reactions to COVID-19 signal the end of the American era. "COVID has reduced to tatters the illusion of American exceptionalism," he writes.[2] But the me of late March was not so sure. And between the radio, the hallway chatter, and the continual mutual accusations across nations and factions, the me now of mid-August is not so sure either; not only about whether American exceptionalism has met the end of its illusion, but whether any of these mutual illusions, imaginations, and projections, which at once animate and tear asunder worlds, can quite be said to end or never be the same because of our once-unnamed virus.

Meanwhile, given my own uncertainty, I too try to secure the world by imagining, throwing a sense of virtual similitude into the future. I picture, in turn, all those closest to me, dying alone. I picture myself dying alone. I try to adjust myself to the imminent possibility of any or all or none of this happening. It is a horror and a release. I keep driving.

[Addendum: In an essay on potent childhood memories, Freud describes processes of omission and displacement involved in their creation—especially those that reverberate later in life in spite of their apparent insignificance. Elements of future and past fuse together to produce an impression in-between—a screen memory—at once concealing and revealing; 'telling,' regardless. To contribute to this writing project carries the vague sensation of such a memory in the making. Prompts arrived across the months, calling for another dispatch from that particular moment in pandemic time. What does one say, not say, omit, displace? Responding to the calls, my jottings in this volume, here and below, might be described as a curious practice of not-saying

that which may have occupied me most in those moments, and yet saying something temporally parallel—and not untrue—in its place. In the fog of the present, in which our experiments with real-time documentation produces texts through filters known and unknown to ourselves, only time can help conjure the in/significances of ongoing re-collections.]

Emily Ng

A Week of (Not) Knowing

The second week of March in New York presented a particular set of challenges. On Monday, there were new closures on the West Coast. On Wednesday, the NBA was the first major sports league to cancel games as the WHO declared that COVID-19 had become a pandemic. On Thursday, Tom Hanks and Rita Wilson tested positive—a headline announced, "now everyone knows someone who is infected." Public school attendance in the city fell from normal levels early in the week to 85% on Thursday, and then to 68% on Friday, when the city announced 54 confirmed cases. While local officials deferred announcing decisions about a lockdown, New York City residents had to balance the increasingly undeniable reality of COVID's arrival with a dogged, collective determination to go about life as normal.

In the absence of a definitive order for change, my wife Diana and I clung to our established routines. When our son's daycare shut last minute for a day of deep cleaning on Wednesday, I rushed him to a Bright Horizons back-up center and went to work. On the subway ride home, I sneezed into my hand, and imagined the collective concern of the other passengers on the train. It was the first time that I remember having an overpowering feeling that I should be wearing a mask. And yet, despite a silent promise to buy one soon, I was on the subway unmasked again later that day.

Yet attempts to ignore the virus grew more difficult by the hour. At lunchtime on Wednesday, I left my office without my usual Tupperware container before changing my mind on the stairs to return to the office. While waiting in line at the food truck, I imagined a headline in a newspaper linking this container to a super-spreader event: I decided I would opt for Styrofoam after all. But as I reached the front of the line, the owner reached out and grabbed it from my hand before I could make my request. As I watched him fill it with food, I felt intense regret, wishing I had said something to stop him. The next day, my reckless lunch eating behavior still on my mind, I called in by Zoom to an administrative meeting taking place two floors below my office, a belated attempt to atone for the lack of caution I showed the day before. My behavior reminded me of Sigmund Freud's "Rat Man" patient as I increasingly acted our competing impulses of preserving normalcy and embracing a new set of epidemic-mandated behaviors.[3]

On Saturday the 14th, I decided to take my children to their weekly swimming lesson. At the front desk, the receptionist took our temperature and required we sanitize our hands, first-time COVID experiences for us. While my daughter practiced flutter kicks to the next section of the pool, I waded into the shallow end with my son for a "Parent and Me" class. Only one other father-child pair had showed up in the fully enrolled class. The instructor cheerfully took us through familiar routines—waterfall crossing, edge jump, flotation device lounge, plastic toy chase. The children, in previous weeks eager to participate, cried inconsolably throughout the lesson. Baffled, our swim teacher commented to another staff member, "I don't get it, none of my tricks are working today. It's like they know something we don't." Perhaps almost as distressed as my son, I had been continually questioning my decision to come, the empty locker room and sparsely populated pool serving as irrefutable evidence of my own poor judgment.

As we climb out of the pool, our instructor smiles and says, "See you next week." In the moment, still hours before Mayor Bill de Blasio would announce the closing of schools, bars, and public places in the city, I already knew. We won't be seeing you for a long time.

Nicholas Bartlett

To Be AND Not to Be a Citizen

March 12, 2020, a new message has appeared in my electronic mailbox. It comes from my school's Vice President for Administration, who has been recently entrusted with the new title of COVID-19 Response Team Lead.

I stare at the screen, while a gripping anguish floods my body. The message is addressed to the entire "SLC Community" of students, faculty, and staff, but I feel it speaks to me, as if I am being hailed. "COVID-19 Update: Spring Travel Plans" reads the message's subject heading, providing some hint into the content of the email's text body:

> Dear SLC Community,
>
> As you have likely already seen, last night President Trump announced limitations regarding travel from Europe to the United States. As you have also likely seen, the details of this development are not entirely clear. [...]. At this time, we caution all members of the Sarah Lawrence community of European citizenship about returning home or traveling to Europe for spring break and/or during the College's two weeks of remote/online classes, and recommend either remaining in on-campus housing or at another location within the U.S. Because this travel ban's guidelines could shift at a moment's notice, members of our community would then be unable to return home and/or to campus. [...]

The message hits me like a slap on the face. I try to process the words whereby my college administration seeks to translate the murky oval office address Trump delivered yesterday. This is the first concrete reverberation of the newly enforced travel ban on the micro-ecology of my daily life. I moved to NYC to join the anthropology department at Sarah Lawrence College 11 years ago, but my inner circle lives overseas, in Italy and in Southeast Asia. I was not planning on leaving for spring break, but the announced travel restrictions (due to become effective in less than 48 hours) strike at the heart of my transnational constellation of affections. I suddenly become aware of an emotional reality that was hiding in plain sight: my own world-system is predicated on the fantasy of being able to go home, if I need to.

When non-immigrants try to imagine or discuss the bureaucratic ordeal of obtaining a temporary work visa or a permanent resident status, they often forget that immigrants do not only want to get in; but they also want to be able to *get out*, for migration concerns the right and desire to both leave and return to one's own country.

When, after six years spent in purgatory wait, I finally received my green card on the eve of a long-awaited sabbatical, I discovered that to preserve my new permanent resident status I should avoid leaving the US for extended periods of time. I had thought the green card was the end of the restrictions that came with my previous H1-B work visa, but I was wrong: "No, you will not be able to be away doing fieldwork for nine months," my immigration attorney's words left me dizzy and speechless. "I know it is absurd," she added, trying to infuse some compassion in her explanation, "but the idea behind it is that you want to be in the U.S. on a permanent basis. If you go away for months, you run the risk of getting charged with abandonment and have your green card confiscated at a U.S. point of entry."

There is a double ethnocentrism in conventional representations of human mobility. It's not only that the US and Western Europe are generally imagined as the only destinations of migratory flows from the Global South; the focus is generally placed on people's aspiration to get in, as if the need to return or to go back and forth did not matter. Within these destination-centric models of migration, the desire for homecoming is either neglected or dismissed as a privilege for a few.

On the same day that the World Health Organization upgraded the novel coronavirus outbreak to the status of a global pandemic and Italy proclaimed a nation-wide lockdown, Trump announced sweeping travel restriction on Europe:

> At the very start of the outbreak, we instituted sweeping travel restrictions on China [...]. The European Union failed to take the same precautions and restrict travel from China and other hotspots. As a result, a large number of new clusters in the United States were seeded by travelers from Europe. To keep new cases from entering our shores, we will be suspending all travel from Europe to the United States for the next 30 days. [...]. There will be exemptions for Americans who have undergone appropriate screenings, and these prohibitions will not only apply to the tremendous amount of trade and cargo, but various other things as we get approval. Anything coming from Europe to the United States is what we are discussing.[4]

Hours later, the President of my HDFC co-op building in Harlem texted me to ask me about my whereabouts and make sure I was not planning on receiving visitors from Europe or Italy, where he knows I come from. On the eve of these presidential communications, my partner was supposed to embark on a 26-hour flight to come visit me from Singapore, where he works and lives. As the events unfolded, we decided it was safer that he cancel his travel plans. It was a painful decision to take. We knew we were never going to meet again in the world we used to know. "By the time you land in NYC, rules could have changed again," I had told him, worried about his seemingly endlessness flight. "Will they realize that I am actually coming from Singapore once I go through passport control?" he responded hinting at the possible consequences of trying to enter the US with an Italian passport.

Unlike Singapore, for which no travel warning had been issued, Italy had suddenly become a Level 3 country. The CDC (i.e., the Centers for Disease Control) had issued a Travel Health Notice urging Americans to avoid all nonessential travel to Italy and a Level 4 "Do Not Travel" warning for the northern regions of Lombardy and Veneto.[5] As my partner and I speak over a 13-hour-time-difference, we try to rehearse the familiar passport check drill. As citizens of Italy who travel often, we have both gone through it countless times, but now we are unable to determine whether possession of a Singapore airlines boarding pass will constitute enough evidence of personal non-contamination. "Even if they saw that you just landed from Singapore," I asked my partner, "how would you prove that you have actually been in Singapore for the past two months and have had no exposure to the cluster outbreaks in Italy?" Rather than travel documents granting safe passage in a foreign land, passports are now transformed into clues of the individual's possible contamination.

Earlier on, at the beginning of the year, during another political crisis that now seemed forgotten, several American citizens of Iranian descent had been stopped at the border.[6] The blatant violation of constitutional rights—gone largely unnoticed among most of my American acquaintances and friends—had disconcerted me. Perhaps I was oversensitive because I was about to re-enter the US after a long research leave overseas and I was terrified that my green card could be revoked. "Yes, I have been away for more than 180 days," I had admitted to the Border Patrol Officer at JFK Airport. He had informed me that this constituted grounds for losing my permanent resident status, but eventually he decided to grace me. "For this one time," he said, "I'll let you go." I had been lucky, but after the early January temporary detention of American citizens of Iranian descent returning from a ski trip to Canada, it had become clear that border crossing was an increasingly uncertain affair. "Anything now is possible," I had thought. But this time, reality has clearly surpassed my border-crossing paranoia.

Trump's televised address disseminated panic and confusion. It was not clear who qualified as "American": citizens? Permanent residents? What type of exemptions? What type of screenings? To take place where? EU leaders complained that the decision had been taken unilaterally, not just without consulting them, but also without informing them. Meanwhile, travelers scrambled to understand the extent of the ban. In the following hours, international airports across the Atlantic were either deserted or jammed. Passengers already at the gate and ready to board had to take snap decisions on whether to cancel or fly anyway. Major US airports emptied out, while a frantic crowd of escaping Americans invaded European hubs.

Since the 2016 presidential election in the US, the administration of the liberal arts institution where I work has often expressed open disagreement vis-à-vis Trump's policies. Not this time. I reread the Vice-President's message that popped up in my mailbox: "Here we go," I think to myself, "I am trapped."

Trump is not my President. Not because I did not vote for him, but because I cannot vote.

"You do not miss much, anyway," joke my American friends when I remind them that, as a permanent resident, I am not allowed to vote in any US elections. I say similar things to immigrants living in Italy who complain about their nonvoting status: "Italian electoral politics is pathetic, you do not miss much." "We are in the same boat," I often tell them. As an Italian citizen residing abroad, I cannot vote in municipal and regional administrative elections; as a resident in the United States, I cannot vote in the election for the European parliament, while as far as national political elections go, I only can choose from a very limited set of unconvincing characters running for the overseas constituency.

I have never given much thought to my exclusion from US electoral privileges, or to the erosion of my voting prerogatives in Italy, never, until now. Would I feel less helpless if I could cast my vote? I feel hostage of incompetent people, expropriated of the illusion of having even a modicum of agency over their mandate.

"Americans pay as much as $20,000 for last-minute flights," tweeted a *New York Times* reporter from Charles de Gaulle airport in Paris, on the day after Trump's announced travel ban.[7] A series of additional guidelines on the screenings and exemptions for Americans were later released by the White House, which explained that the ban only applied to foreign nationals and that Americans and permanent residents were to "be directed to a limited number of airports where screening can take place." But the ban had already spun out of control, severely impacting the actual availability of flights. In a frantic attempt to contain financial losses, airline carriers began to cancel flights, further fueling the panic wave. Over the weekend, images from Chicago O'Hare International airport showed thousands of travelers returning from Europe trapped in closed quarters, waiting in line for hours as the virus spread on. They portrayed an indistinguishable

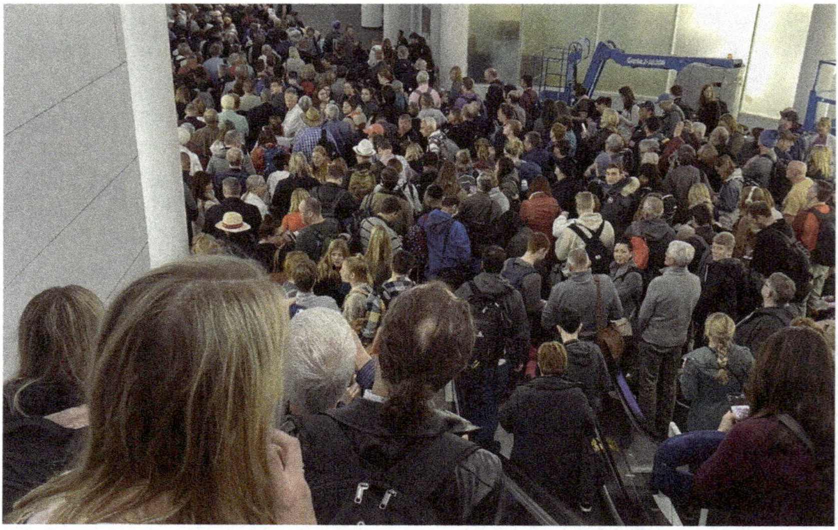

Fig. 1.3 A field ripe for viral transmission, O'Hare Airport, Chicago, March 15, 2020. (Photo courtesy of Brooke Geiger McDonald/Twitter)

crowd of humans seeking individual salvation and possibly getting infected while waiting in line to undergo health checks (Fig. 1.3).[8]

Like Benjamin's dialectical images that emerge in a flash,[9] these travelers' snapshots expose with unprecedented force the contradictions of citizenship and its exclusionary apparatus, the paradoxes of shutting down borders on the very day the belated declaration of a state of pandemic had revealed there was no longer an outside to the contagion. Conjuring claustrophobic visions of the danger from within, these photographic records unveil the oxymoron of homeland security, blasting any illusion of domestic safety.

Aurora Donzelli

Virtual Mourning, Virtual Loss

In early April 2020, I received a message via WhatsApp, an instant messaging service popular among Indonesians, that my great uncle had died after complaining about *sesak napas*, "shortness of breath." In its Indonesian context, *sesak napas* or "shortness of breath" is a common way to describe respiratory discomfort among the elderly. At the same time, *sesak napas* is a phrase that appears frequently in obituaries, often in one or two sentences that describe a probable cause of death. These utterances and turns of phrases in obituaries and text messages are key in my own experiences of the COVID-19 pandemic, especially in how the pandemic changes mourning and remembrance. At a time when death and mourning are not accompanied by the warmth of physical co-presence, I experienced virtual sociality as solidarity at a time of loss.

I never knew what the official cause of death for my great uncle was, but it seemed like a form of unanticipated death that was all too common in the early weeks of the COVID-19 pandemic. True, he was 93 years old, and it could have been his lifelong habit of smoking from a tobacco pipe, or it could have been an unexpected bout of pneumonia. And yet, at a time when the world suddenly pays attention to respiratory ailments and how they might change lives all of a sudden, this felt to me like a death that signaled the end of an era of a generation of elders.

In a series of messages from my own family, I received WhatsApp videos of a burial procession with soldiers wearing masks, and a large tent in the middle of a military cemetery, where my great uncle was buried with the military honors that are customarily provided to war veterans in Indonesia. Like his siblings, who fought in the Indonesian War of Independence, he was given a military salute, and mourners sat in rows of chairs put under tents that sheltered them from the tropical sun. This time, however, something was different. Everyone, including the pallbearers, wore masks to cover their mouths and noses, and, instead of huddling close together, mourners distanced themselves from one another, leaving one or two chairs between one another. More surprising, however, was that I noticed an absence of many older relatives and kin who would have otherwise been present at such a funeral. Among Indonesian families, presence at a funeral is almost certainly expected for both kin and friends, and yet, at the same time, the absence of my older relatives at this funeral was more than understandable. At this point, both the Indonesian government and national media outlets extensively reported on how COVID-19 is particularly dangerous for the elderly.

Death and burials feel like a quotidian matter of life in Indonesia, especially in its rural areas, where wakes involve one's neighbors, families, and kin coming from out of town and even from abroad. A large number of mourners seem to signify the greatness of the departed, and one might say that the departed bring families closer together than ever before. My own grandfather's death, for instance, was remembered by many as when "we had to rent two buses for all the mourners." And yet, at the same time, the pandemic presents an incredible irony that negates all of these customs—one should not gather in large numbers, especially after deaths that might be caused by the coronavirus. Even in this funeral video on WhatsApp, the soldiers who marched along with the pallbearers were generously distanced from another, leaving a generous amount of space for everyone to see my great uncle's flag-draped coffin.

In urban Java, where I spent my childhood and my early years of adulthood, death is a profoundly social affair. Rather than the slogan of "respect for privacy," which I find to be common in American contexts, Javanese Indonesians attend the funerals of distant relatives and acquaintances alike. The bereaved, to them, need the company of others to face grief, although many admit that painful moments of emotional distress usually come after visiting mourners have left. In Kupang, the field site of my dissertation research in eastern Indonesia, deaths are an even more elaborate affair. Entire offices would take a day off to pay respects to the deceased kin of a coworker, and one would customarily bring an envelope with some cash in it to help the bereaved cover the cost of funeral-related rituals and feasts.

For Indonesians, mourning is rarely a solitary experience—one says goodbye to the departed in the company of many others. And yet, because of the pandemic, the death of a relative turned into a moment of virtual mourning for me—one that I experienced primarily through the instant messages and Facebook posts created by others. I read repetitions after repetitions of the same expressions of mourning that Indonesians use, *turut berduka cita* ("I mourn together with you"). Though they are only letters on a screen, the warmth of these words felt like the comforting embraces after a funeral.

Rafadi Hakim

Déjà vu

April 11, 2020. Italy has been in lockdown for more than a month now and the number of deaths is increasing exponentially. Our university, in Upstate New York, decided to close our campus on March 19, 2020, and to have us teach online. Of course, I knew it was going to happen. In Northern Italy they closed all schools and universities in early March.

When I was talking about this with some of my friends, they just stared at me, dumbfounded. Their eyes were distracted, far away from mine. Mine had been in tears the night before. What will happen next? Northern Italy is in a very bad situation right now. The virus started, and spread very rapidly, in two regions: Lombardy and Veneto. My family lives in the latter. My parents are old, my brother suffers from a very rare form of asthma. He was born that way. Nobody has been able to heal him. I can still hear his heavy, whistling breathing while he was asleep. We were happy together, we were kids. I am really worried, this virus is just in the air, anyone can breathe it. And yet nobody seems to care. My anger and disappointment are mixed with senses of guilt because I am far away from my family who might need my assistance and love.

I try to convey my anxiety to my friends and colleagues in the United States:

- "We will close our schools and university pretty soon too. This virus is borderless, it travels long ways, it is very contagious, it is there up in the air, you can breathe it."
- "I think the virus is already here among us," I said once while I was considering whether to take a spinning class in a very small gym fitness room with no windows. I just love spinning so much. It removes my anxieties and refreshes my mind.
- "Oh dear, just take this class with me," a friend of mine said.
- "You don't understand. People need to be distant at least one or two meters. This room is too small to exercise altogether. I just can't do it."

I didn't take that class. I'll never be able to take a spinning class in a small room ever again. I am so sad. I wished I had video-recorded one of those classes for a project I am doing on fitness culture. I didn't. It's just part of my memory now.

The spinning instructor wrote to me on Facebook Messenger that night. It was March 6, 2020. He asked me why I was not in his class. I replied to him hastily around midnight:

> [...] My family in Italy (Mom, Dad, and brother) have been going through a very hard time because of this Coronavirus. As for today, there are almost 4,000 people infected, 150 deaths and the majority is in the area where my family lives. These numbers have been going up at an unprecedented speed.

> My parents are old and they have some health issues, so I am extremely worried. You might wonder: "What does this have to do with spinning?" Well, I've been following all this very closely and I think that the room in which we spin is NOT safe for participants, but only for the instructor. Our bikes are too close to each other—the safe distance being at least 1 meter from each other (they are keeping people at 2 meters right now in Italy). I can breathe other people's breaths while I spin if someone is sitting next to me. While this is fine in normal times, I don't think I can have this in a time in which everyone is starting to panic about this virus which is transmittable via droplets (coughs, sneezes, or simply breadths—if it gets to your eyes, nose or mouth, of course). In Italy, they have prohibited the handshake and any other kind of salutation in which touch is involved, and they keep people at two meters of distance. Ideally, it would be nice to have less bikes and more space in-between bikes in our spinning room. Or, alternatively, one vacant bike next to spinners [...]

Fifteen days later our gym closed. What's happening? Are there going to be dead people here as well? In the meantime, Italy had been put in total lockdown. The entire country. Deaths and infected cases were increasing at an unparalleled and unbelievable rate. Is this a bad dream? I am just worried.

March 22, 2020. Bergamo, one of the northern Italian towns with more deaths in Italy, sends images and videos around the world. "Please help us," beg doctors and nurses in overflowing hospitals. The capacity of hospitals has reached its limits. Military trucks are then used to take the victims, as if it were in wartime, away from these hospitals. The videos that went viral are heartbreaking.[10]

Is this real or is this a war movie? What's happening in Italy? I decide to send those videos to my friend and to my spinning instructor. They still think I am overreacting. They don't really comment on them. They make me feel I am not doing the right thing. Am I wrong?

- "The virus has killed so many people, they need to take the dead bodies away from the hospitals, you see?" I try to explain. "They used military trucks to do so."

I saw my dad crying twice in my life. The second time was when he received the results of his COVID-19 test: negative. I was almost sure he was infected by the virus. He was sure, too. He knew he made the usual mistakes. He risked what he was not supposed to risk. He went to a dinner one night. It was the beginning of the lockdown craziness in Italy. "The dinner was amazing," he said. Twelve participants, out of fourteen, tested positive. He was one of the lucky ones.

– "They are dying like flies," my father said. "Many old people are dying but young people too. I have never seen anything like this. This is not like the flu," he confessed.

The virus is here, I can feel it. It is between and among us. It's just everywhere. It is in my classroom with 90 students. I usually like to teach and walk close to the students, look at them in the eyes, try to see who they are. I like to ask them questions, to make my lectures more fun. Today is the last day of class. I need to say goodbye to my students. I need to tell them that I'll see them through my computer screen. I am very committed to continue to meet their eyes while I lecture. They finally decided to close all schools in New York State. I act quickly. Students should not sit so close to each other. It is déjà vu.

April 29, 2020. Those images from Bergamo are still populating my mind. It has been more than a month now and the situation in Italy has not improved. 700 or even 1,000 deaths a day. It is unprecedented. When will this stop? It has been a nightmare. It will never stop. Humanity is at risk. Especially the more disadvantaged, the poor, the ones who cannot afford any good living or care or even a good quality, protective mask. It is a very sad night. Like in a movie, or déjà vu, on my computer, I see images of dead bodies piled up in trucks in New York City. This is overwhelming. They are not elegantly transported away, like in Bergamo, however. Instead, they are piled up in large and small trucks or minivans waiting to be thrown into mass graves outside the City.[11]

I talked to one of those gym friends the other day while she was delivering a lesson to me as to how important it is to keep a safe distance and to wear a mask. Finally, the news has reached all minds. Now it is up to us. We can perhaps fight this virus altogether.

Sabina M. Perrino

The Viral Sublime

When I fall asleep at night I enter into oblivion. Any dreams are elsewhere. Once I wake, it all comes crashing down again. It's as if news of the virus comes from outside the apartment and glides through the windows along with the morning light. Often I check the news before sitting up in the bed. Holding a smart phone in my hands, I scroll through the headlines of online newspapers, dispatches from New York, India, Great Britain, Hong King, China, Sweden, Singapore, Mexico, you name it. The virus is everywhere. It has entered into all aspects and fault lines of human existence. Travel bans. Overburdened Hospitals. Death in care homes. Isolation and Loneliness. Virtual teaching, schooling at home. Increased rates of drinking and abuse. Health disparities. Unemployment lines and statistics. Unpaid migrant workers stuck far from home.

The virus is also nowhere precise and singular and tangible (Fig. 1.4). I have come to call this the "viral sublime," without any hard thinking on that—sublime in the way that the virus and its effects are at once everywhere and nowhere, and how it exceeds the ability of a single mind to grasp its workings, its spread through the world, the countless ways people's lives and deaths have been affected. Sublime as in inspiring awe, and a correlated

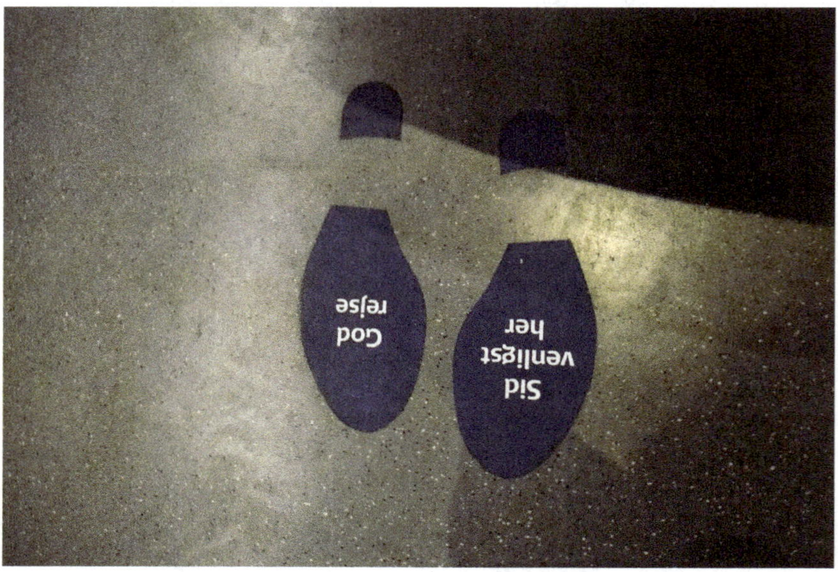

Fig. 1.4 Signs posted on the floor of a metro train, Copenhagen, April 2020. (Photo by R. Desjarlais)

incapacity to comprehend the allness of it. It's impossible to fathom the full extent of its damage, the tolls exacted, its many obscure pathways, or what the near or distant future will bring. While the numbers keep increasing. It's overwhelming—and fascinating, those many interlacing dimensions of a plague. And viral, too, these operations in body and mind. Wavering thoughts and imaginings of the virus move about like the contagion itself, as imagined. *Cytokine storm* is an apt term, medically, and phenomenologically.

"It's madness," writes a friend, far away in space and time.

"What is happening across the globe is so surreal," writes another.

Viral shredding. Self-quarantine. Social distancing. Sheltering in place. Herd immunity. Contact tracing. Corona shaming. Ghost games. Ground glass opacity. These are the idioms of the day, words to live and fret by.

"The virus doesn't care," says a medical anthropologist. Meaning that the virus goes about its viral ways without regard or concern for the worries or strivings of any human beings.

CONFRONT YOUR DISCOMFORT reads a sign made of block letters printed onto sheets of paper and taped to the glass windows of a nearby shop (Fig. 1.5).

Robert Desjarlais

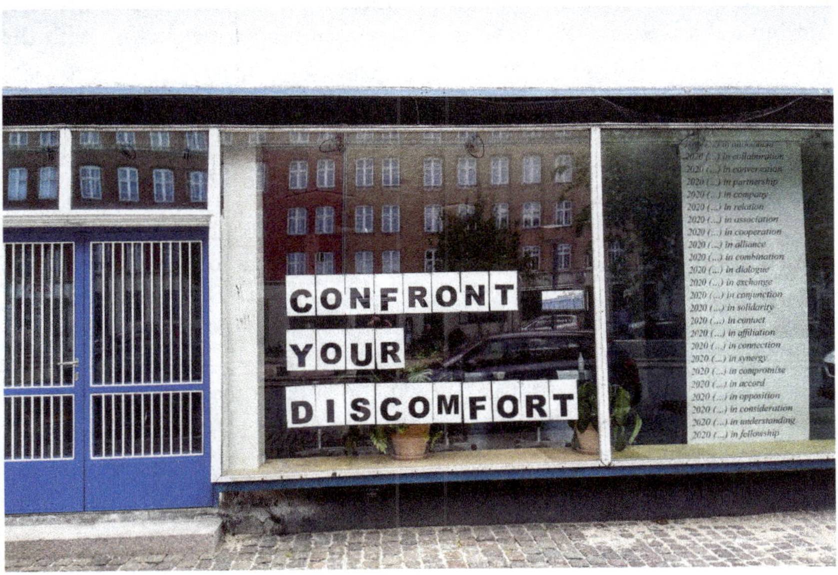

Fig. 1.5 Sign on the window of an office, closed during the pandemic, Copenhagen, April 2020. (Photo by R. Desjarlais)

Anger

I know I hit the fucking button, but it didn't matter because my opponent must have done so first. Maybe they tapped their "charge attack" milliseconds before I did, maybe we tapped it at the exact same time and the machine had to make a choice about who would get to go first. It didn't much matter because in this case it meant I lost and someone else won. My last Pokemon was down to very little strength as it was, its bar of energy or "CP" (combat power) down to the last fifth, and therefore colored red. This meant any hit from a charge attack would defeat it, no matter the match-up or how effective the specific attack. My opponent was some anonymous person I would likely never be matched up with again, since the process is completely random and tens of millions of people play on a regular basis, worldwide. I was one of them, had been for a year. I'd caught over 10,000 Pokemon, evolved hundreds, hatched as many eggs and given as many gifts to "Friends," and I had a Pokedex with very rare Pokemon I'd won in raids or through accomplished missions. I'd been battling other players a lot lately, trapped inside much of the day and unable to catch more Pokemon or spin Pokestops on walks.

All of that effort put into this game and it all comes down to that one instance of smart phone–human (non)interaction, a disregard of my having pushed a button, after having done so countless times before with the desired effect. That non-event, what would have been, should have been the translation of minor haptic energy into game action—one subtle finger tap into a Roserade's high powered solar beam attack. Instead, this my last Pokemon was defeated and I was the official loser of the match. The game wouldn't dare make such a claim, instead showing my avatar clapping with no expression as the words "Good Effort" appear. If this is an attempt to calm me down, to lessen the explosion of rage that builds inside of me when I play this game lately, then it failed as much as I just had. Dismally. I feel that anger build and build until I think how good it would feel to hurl my phone across the room and against the far wall. Such release to see the phone come apart, splitting down the side along the visible crease, revealing the innards of the hateful thing.

But I can't do that, I can't explain that feeling of destructive joy to my wife the next day. I could not have this conversation:

"What the hell happened to your phone?"
"Oh, that. I was playing Pokemon Go last night and I was in battle mode..."
"What?"
"I was competing to defeat the three Pokemon that some random person chose against my three that I chose, and I lost."
"And why did that upset you so much?"
"Well, I had been playing really well, I had gotten up to the rank of over 1700 for the first time in the lesser league. I had settled on three that were really good against most competition and was winning all sorts of extra awards, mostly stardust and Pokemon candy so I could evolve Pokemon and make them stronger."
"Ok..."
"Anyway, it's Ultra League play now, that changed abruptly yesterday and so now you can pick any three so long as they do not have a CP greater than 2500. The previous league was limited to Pokemon with a CP of 1500, so the strategy is a lot different..."
"I do not give a shit, do not throw away money on a stupid game please."

I wasn't just upset about one loss. I've lost slightly more battles than I've won, overall, after playing over 2000 of them since February.

"Why are you playing so often?" I ask myself. I cannot have that conversation.

What pissed me off, what still pisses me off, if I think about it too much, is the amount of effort I knew it would take to stop losing. It took a lot of losing to figure out which three Pokemon to use in the previous league, but this league was different. People were using different Pokemon whose weaknesses and attacks I didn't know as well. I also didn't know my Pokemon at that rank of CP either. In battles, you don't have the option to change the Pokemon you are using from the three you pick, not before seeing those of your opponents. And you are swiftly punished if you choose wrong. From the opening, if your opponent is a species that your species of Pokemon is especially vulnerable to (e.g., grass beats ground and water), you could end up defeated after a handful of fast attacks. If you switch to another of your three before that one is defeated, and you choose wrong in a panic or out of ignorance, then you could have a second Pokemon knocked out with no escape (since a thirty-second timer prevents you from swapping for your third Pokemon right away). You can even have a decent or even matchup and then the charge attack of your opponent fills up at astonishing speed. Every charge attack takes time to "charge" while you lob fast attacks, but some refill after only three fast attacks and some take a dozen or more. That disparity can force you to use one of your two shields in quick succession, leaving you unprotected as the battle rages on and your opponent levels charged attacks at you that you can't defend against.

I didn't know all of this before the Pandemic.

Figuring all of this out, the species, their attacks, their weaknesses, and multiplying that by the hundreds of possible Pokemon that any player can catch and use, times the order you should use them in... all of that leads to exponential calculations that, coupled with quick decision-making, can lead to disastrous results. It can also fill you with adrenaline and excitement when it goes against you or in your favor. (Desjarlais talks about this in similar ways about "blitz chess" play in his book *Counterplay*. But I don't remember him ever throwing a chess board across a room).[12]

"Fine, but why do you get so upset you want to scream and break things?"

I cannot have that conversation. I could not have that conversation with my wife, or with anyone who didn't play, mostly because, while I might be able to account for the specific actions, the phone, its destruction, in that moment, it could not come close to accounting for my anger, for my feeling I could boil over at any moment. For my desire to let out a primal scream, right now, right this second at no one and nothing.

Most concerning to me isn't that I might damage my phone or annoy my wife, but what happens as a result of the reaction that I do let myself have, not throwing my phone but instead raising my voice in frustration, after I lost. When I do this, my nearby, disabled son reacts by standing up suddenly and proceeding to the restroom, assuming, it would appear, that I am annoyed at him for not going. That has also happened at times, late at night, a normal part of our ritual as I care for him and try to avoid him wetting himself.

"Surely that's what's upsetting you, really! I mean, it must be so hard to take care of a thirteen, soon to be fourteen-year-old son at one in the morning and constantly worried he might soil himself. Or maybe it is all the additional childcare you are doing as a result of the Pandemic. That combined with economic disaster, police violence, social unrest…"

No. It's the game, it's my phone. I delete the Pokemon Go app, the fourth time in as many months, and I apologize to my son.

Josh Reno

Flickers of Ordinariness

It is a sunny late morning in Milan. May is drawing to an end as I ride on the back of my father's BMW Enduro motorbike. My father and I are running ordinary errands—as we usually do when I come home for my extended late spring visits, from NYC. The bike is a convenient way to navigate Milan's congestion-riddled streets where parking—as is the case in many Italian cities—has become almost impossible. While riding on the bike, seated behind my father, I scan the streets' everyday life and catch glimpses of new ways of attending to things.

The city has begun loosening the lockdown less than two weeks ago.[13] Restaurants and cafes have re-opened—though supposedly only for take-out service. Salons, stores, and barbershops are also finally back in business, but with a new modus operandi: a client's temperature is taken upon arrival, and a rigid regime of appointments is in place to avoid servicing more than one customer at once. Vivid yellow, bright white, electric green, or flashy red-hued stencils have been placed on the asphalt in proximity of bus stops, stores, and even kiosks where lines of humans are likely to form. "STAY HERE" loudly hail the colorful markings on the asphalt. They address foot-travelers with a new form of disciplinary interpellation. Sometimes they use Italian/English bilingual wording ("*stai qui*/stand here"), sometimes just Italian ("*attendi qui*"), and sometimes they resort to iconic signs, which are believed to be more universally decodable: rows of aligned and properly distanced white footprints pave the space in front of Giannasi—an historic roasted-chicken kiosk in Milan. I notice how people compliantly wait for their turn, making sure their feet are positioned exactly on the white footprints.

How the virus actually spreads is still a scientific mystery. Is it airborne or does it only travel through the droplets spread by someone's infectious sneezes or coughs? Some studies have proposed a correlation between the spread of the contagion and air pollution, suggesting the virus does not only travel through the droplets but rather attaches itself to pollution particles, sticking in the air well after the infected human's passage. Is a six-foot distance enough to prevent us from inhaling the droplets? Can the virus linger in the air and persist in aerosol form? Will the Plexiglas barriers now being installed in grocery stores and pharmacies over the world be enough to protect those who work there from the lethal droplets? How long can the virus survive on hard surfaces? Can traces of coronavirus stick to the soles of our shoes?[14] What about water? "Traces of coronavirus have been found in Paris's non-drinking water," a news agency reported in mid-April. So far, experts over the world have offered contradictory theories and guidelines. What seems certain is that improvisation is no longer an option in the choreography of contemporary pedestrian movement. Without a definite answer on social distancing effectiveness, people's compliance with the directions uttered by the sidewalk signs responds to a new moral code of both civic conduct and hopeful self-preservation.

The implementation of social distancing rules has created a novel space of moral reasoning and a whole new political economy of service encounters. Practices that were once obvious and natural have now become the object of great scrutiny. What is the proper way to wash one's hands? How goes the walking? How are we supposed to turn our bodies without coming too close to someone walking behind us? There is a new grammar for social and commercial transactions. A new awareness of our bodily presence has kicked in, affecting some more than others, but nonetheless pervasively restructuring ordinary forms of life. Word has it that the handshake—a greeting practice whose earliest representation allegedly dates back to the fifth century BC—may be doomed to disappear. My friend Cristiana, who landed a few days ago in Milan, after a days-long multi-stop journey from California, was taken aback with surprise when her nephew in an audacious display of irreverent affection hugged her. "I realized no one had touched me in three months," she told me. People wonder whether hugs will ever come back and debate about the potential loss of entrenched forms of sociality, which date back to Ancient Greece (Fig. 1.6).

In these somewhat erudite somewhat ordinary discussions, the temporal references associated with Before Christ and Before COVID become blurry, in a time warp of sorts. The semantic play on the double meaning of the acronym BC has become a popular trope in today's mediascape.

I close my eyes, letting the rays of sunshine caress my pale post-lockdown skin. As I am being driven through the streets of my hometown, I lull myself in the illusion that nothing ever happened, that we are not

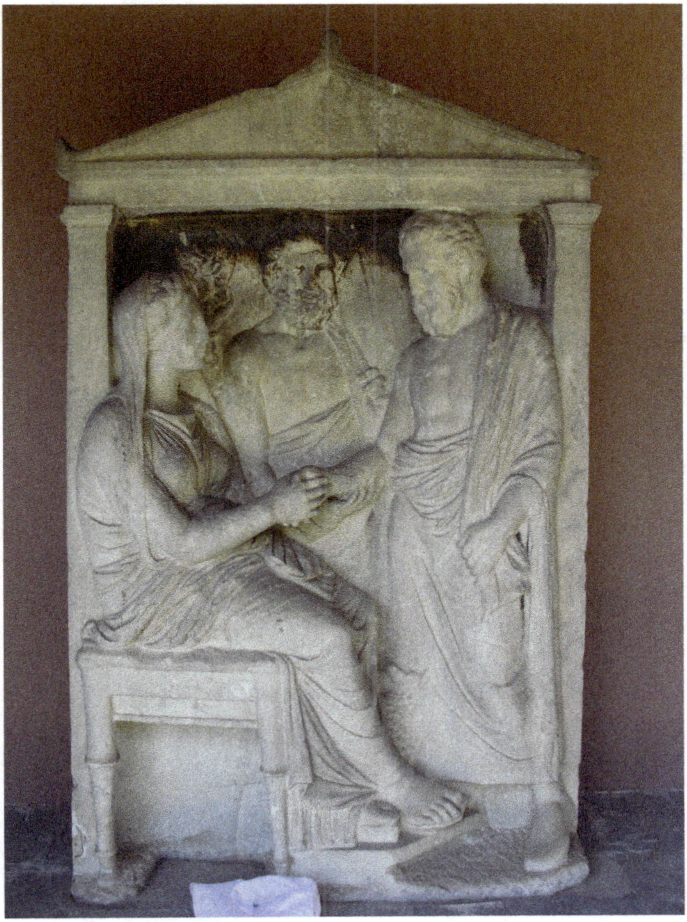

Fig. 1.6 One of the allegedly most ancient representation of the handshake—detail from the grave of Agathon and Sosykrates, Cloister of the Kerameikos Archaeological Museum (Athens). Photo by Tilemahos Efthimiadis, Wikimedia Commons

inhabiting an aftermath; a time "post-." The eerily spectral vistas of the city's deserted streets are gone, and now even their memory is fading in the background, perhaps ousted away by the familiar experience of a morning bike ride in my hometown, driven by my father as I used to be driven since I was a child. For a moment, I seem to be able to retrieve the possibility of just being in the moment, a moment in time open to an unforeseeable future—an openness unrestricted by the unnerving wait for the daily bulletin on the COVID death toll, or the government's Facebook live update on whether and when we could travel again outside our region, visit friends and significant others who are not kin, exercise outdoors, walk in a park, bring the dog out for a walk beyond the enforced limit of 200 meters from one's certified residence. But as soon as I open my eyes, the sight of face masks that everyone in Milan zealously wears reminds me of the planetary trauma that has marked our ordinary lives.

There is a hopefulness of sorts in the temporal prefix "post-" that is now being attached to many noun-phrases: "post-pandemic task force," "post-pandemic age," "post-pandemic world," "post-pandemic travel"—the hope that the pandemic is behind us, the hope that there will not be a second deadlier wave. Newspapers headings reporting epidemiologists and virologists' words constantly remind us of the likelihood of a second wave. This is how pandemics have unfolded in human history. There *is* going to be a second wave, and perhaps even a third. But in spite of its undeniable coefficient of hopefulness, there is an aura of tragedy lingering in the semantics of "post-ness:" the collective awareness that life is now divided between a "before" and an "after."

I close my eyes again, feeling the intensity of my longing for a time before the time of the "post-." It seems incredible that that time was only a few months ago, for it feels as far away as the time of my childhood in Milan.

Aurora Donzelli

Microphantasms of the Pandemic

The apartment where I am residing, in the Vesterbro neighborhood of Copenhagen, seems safe. There is the phantasm of safety, at least, for I feel a sense of security and apartness when I return home after being outside. The door locks tight, and once I take off my coat, gloves, and wash my hands I feel that this space keeps me free of any contaminants, for as long as I remain there. But who knows. It could be around here, somewhere. On the kitchen counter, perhaps, or seeded onto the set of keys I carry with me. Unseen pathogens might have snuck in with me when I returned home after getting coffee this morning—I had forgotten to wash my hands straight off. I only thought of that after taking a few sips from a paper cup. Nothing is clear.

I look out my window quite often and see people across the way, similarly hunkered down, couched within their own peripheral knowings. I try to imagine what their days are like, what's on their minds just then. On slight occasions we see each from afar but we never acknowledge the other's presence.

It's like the city is composed of a thousand peripheral knowings. There's much more than that, actually, in the world at large. Everyone has a slight side view and partial grasp of what's involved as they try to find their way. In these zones of uncertainty, in emergent time, no one anywhere has a clear and comprehensive sense of what's going on. Everyone is in their own little zoom quadrant of knowledge and perception (Fig. 1.7). Each day brings new moments of unlearning, not-knowing, and epistemological and ontological limits. Systems of medical care, knowledge, technology, commerce, and power are fraying at the edges. The center is not holding. Non-mastery, indeed. I doubt that anyone truly feels that they

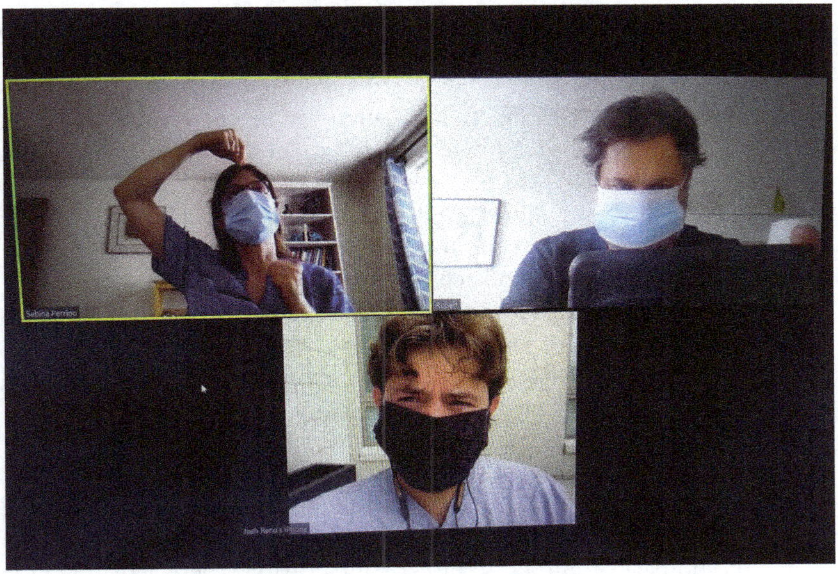

Fig. 1.7 Zoom conversation, with a trying on of masks. April 2020. (Photo by R. Desjarlais)

are a master of everything or anything just now. No masters of the universe, as in decades past. Any precise sense of mastery is an illusion. And yet one still strives for it, in small moments, of writing, knitting, crafting, making, walking, talking, reading, drinking, or watching films that stream into the solitude of one's nights.

Across the way there are children playing in a playground, kicking a ball around, and a child's first steps, her mother walking closely, proudly, behind. Small moments of grace. And then there's the Nordic sunlight, soft, clear and subtle, gaining in strength each day.

To which I would add the gentle encouragement, seek out the phantasmal, trace out its spectral workings and haunting reverberations, tend to the micro-phantasms that thread through everyday life. I return to certain peripheral moments that have captured my own thoughts and imaginings of late.

-as with that afternoon hour, in one of the first day of the shutdown, while I walked along a sidewalk in Vesterbro: I watched as a young man delicately removed his bank card from a telling machine and, with precise gestures with his fingers, wiped down each side and surface of the card with a snow-white cloth.

-or in those first days after the university and other places had closed, but a few cafes were still open: I would go there in mornings to work, with others doing much the same while seated a few meters apart away, each of us going about our tasks while, it seemed, we all knew we were doing something slightly transgressive, and risky.

-or that day when I read about some expert's research study of the slight but altogether significant wind currents that swirl about in the wake of someone walking past or running nearby; since then, when I walk in any of the city's streets, trying to keep the proper distance from others, I try to calculate, with no actual sense of precise calculations, how the virus might circulate in the air swirling past that healthy-looking jogger who just ran by me, or the couple that walked too close to my own two-metered space in the city, the air between us all too transparent.

-or the other morning, as I set out for a walk: while standing at a street corner, waiting for the signal to turn green, I noticed a man across the way, his body decked out in gloves, winter scarf, jacket with the hood pulled over his head, and a mask and dark sunglasses that hid his face, as if he wanted no part of himself in direct contact with others, which led me to wonder—and wonder only—what concerns led him to protect himself so fully.

-or the empty packets of paracetamol tablets I found one day while cleaning the apartment; they were hidden underneath a counter, the once-there contents of which led me to wonder if the previous tenant of the flat had suddenly come down with a fever and, worried for her health and safety, had quickly returned to a family home in another land.

-or of how one can go without thinking about the pandemic for hours at a time, while engaged with some task, and then awareness of its cruel force quickly slips back into consciousness; it's surprising to find that one can actually forget about it for a while, while feeling guilty for having done so.

-or the planes of diffusion that can emerge when one is on one's own for several days at a stretch, and coordinates of time and space, selfhood and language start to lose their bounded tightness and one risks falling into a fugue of crumpled subjectivity and unmade beds.

-and then to step outside and suddenly talk with another living being, in person, in a three-dimensional flow of time beyond the facade of a computer screen, this can almost be like a religious experience, a visceral encounter with the vital presence of another. Somehow, it's the eyes of the other that are most alive.

Robert Desjarlais

Memento mori

May 2020

Time is new. It has a different texture. It is hard to settle down now, hard to read, hard to be silent and still amidst all the silence and stillness jangling and shuffling around.

To tame time, I make detailed schedules, every hour accounted for and punctuated by push-ups—like a scientist in Antarctica. From 11:15 to 12:30 I will write you. Then I will do 15 push-ups. I have been doing push-ups for three weeks but I am not getting stronger. The tree outside my apartment window begins to bud but I do not change.

Always the primordial shock of spring when barren trees come to life again. Barren is a word reserved for trees and women. "Barren" is a word I learned reading as a kid. I heaped it in with "consumption" and "paroxysm"—pains and afflictions of earlier centuries having nothing to do with modern flesh, with my body. "Quarantine" also fell into this category.

Yet, here I find myself. Nothing much comes from these quarantine hours. I work relentlessly, twelve, fourteen hours a day, zoom meetings and google docs, track changes and slack channels, but when I lie down at night, I can't think of what I've accomplished. These days are broad dead fields. The Romans sowed the fields of their enemies with salt. We too have been conquered, though we still stoop to sow. The chia seeds that I faithfully mist do not sprout, the sourdough starter begins to mold along the edges, failing to catch the right wild yeast. Dead days. But also days of the dead. Days where people are suffering and dying, just over there. Out of sight.

I always wondered about this in my research, how there could be mass graves on the edge of town while the markets in the central square sold oranges. Now I think I understand better. You keep pushing life—keep washing spoons, calling your brother, writing emails, peeling oranges—but how also, all the time, the dread hovers.

Anyone could be the one. Contagion sneaks around, like informants, like spies. "We are all connected." This used to sound like pablum. Now we reckon with its material truth, its vectors, surfaces, economies. We exchange droplets, aerosol, immunity, rumors, advice, admonishment. Emotions are also contagious. We exchange fear. We trade recklessness.

Even so. Still. Go on. Do 15 push-ups. Do them on your knees. Do them with trembling arms. Do them because you need to be stronger now.

In the middle of the world's catastrophe, it is perverse to dwell on small desires and disappointments. Nevertheless, I am annoyed by a colleague on a zoom call. I am bored of the lentil soup I have made. I wish for pleasures, entertainments, distractions. The petty and insignificant stick to the catastrophic, as an insect sticks her eggs to an oak tree with larval glue.

I should not be restless. I should not be bored. In these incarcerated hours, I should count my blessings. Be grateful I have a job, a roof over my head, an internet connection. Be grateful I draw breath.

Before everything shut down, instructions for handwashing began to pop-up everywhere. In the restroom at my office, a poster illustrated the correct protocol. "Washing your hands properly takes about as much time as singing Happy Birthday twice," we were advised. "Apply enough soap," we were warned. "Rub hands palm to palm," we were cautioned. The final step in the ritual promised: "And your hands are safe," with a drawing of uplifted palms, as if in prayer.

"A memento mori is an artwork designed to remind the viewer of their mortality and of the shortness and fragility of human life" the Tate museum website tells me. "Remember death" or "remember that you have to die." I scroll through dancing skeletons, maidens and reapers clasping hands, death holding a rake or a broom, fluttering candles, rotting peaches and oranges, skulls, the lost beloved's hair braided in a silver locket.

Curious fact: it was only in the aftermath of the black plague that women became writers. What new understanding of death and fragility will emerge after this? What silence will become unbearable?

Memento mori: wash your hands and sing happy birthday twice.

And your hands are safe.

Dirty hands. Scratching your nose. Not looking both ways. Braking too slow. A soldier offended. A stumble on the stairs. A cough in an elevator. The difference between life and death can be small, random, an accident, a joke.

Alexa Hagerty

Legislative Intimacies

—"*Ciao, come ti butta la fase 2 bis?*" ("Hi there, how is phase 2 bis treating you?")

—"*Ciao ! Io continuo con la fase 1 per altri sei mesi, non è poi cosí male…*" ("Hi! I am staying put in phase 1 for six more months. I am starting to like it").[15]

Although Italy's Phase 2 officially began in early May with a so-called soft opening, it was only after a second round of executive measures issued in mid-May[16] (commonly referred to as "Phase 2 bis") that people were able to see friends again and leave their houses without having to fill in a legally binding self-certification—provided by the Ministry of Homeland Security (*Ministero degli Interni*)—stating the purpose of their outing. Most of my friends, however, seem still unwilling or incapable of abandoning the reclusive regime of the previous two months.

I take a second look at the message that has appeared on my iPhone's display, uncertain whether to interpret my friend's response as a preemptive rejection of my potential invitation to meet or as description of his actual disposition to the world. His proclaimed clinging to phase 1 does not surprise me. I feel much the same way. Curled up in a state of comfortable numbness, I am desireless and oblivious to the small pleasures that I once held dear. I forgot when and how I began to embrace this new self-withdrawn version of myself. But I recall some gradualness in my metamorphosis. It felt like a slow-motion fall into a bottomless void. It was painful and unnerving, but gradual. And the deeper I would fall, the more numb I would become, until I was enwrapped in a thick crusty cocoon. What is this new crust? Is it a mutation of my own skin? Is it an emotional reverberation of the surgical gloves and face mask I have to wear? Is it a still uncharted symptom of the mysterious infection? It would not be surprising, for the virus has been scientifically proven to affect our sensorium in uncanny ways. Scientists now agree that loss of smell and taste are to be added to the official list of symptoms for COVID-19.

When we first heard about the enforcement of draconian lockdown measures in the Wuhan region of China, we thought the resolution was archaic—a medieval or early modern response that appeared somewhat anachronistic for the third millennium. TV screens and digital devices conjured imageries of a dystopian future mixed with medieval visions of the Apocalypse. A vertigo of sorts took hold as we watched scenes that seemed to concern an elsewhere, or perhaps a distant future or a remote past. Only a few weeks later, however, Italy embarked on what turned out to be the first world's nation-wide lockdown of the COVID era. With physical isolation as the seemingly only remedy to stop the exponential growth of the contagion, the state adopted unprecedented legislation. Between the end of February and the beginning of March, a rapid succession of executive measures spawned in a viral progression that mirrored that of the contagion. As the infections spiked up, more restrictions were implemented. As days went by, more and more areas went into lockdown and more and more activities were suspended. By March 11, all civil and religious ceremonies, including funerals, were banned; schools, universities, stores, gyms, cinemas, theaters, and museums were closed. A 6 pm curfew on bars and restaurants was enforced, while private and public companies were invited to suspend their activities and place all non-essential workers on leave.[17]

The nation-wide lockdown established by the executive decree of March 11 stands out as the most severe set of measures ever imposed since World War II. In the attempt to make the restrictions less unpopular, the government deliberately turned the name of the decree into a hashtag, officially calling it *Decreto #IoRestoaCasa* (#IStayHome Decree). The decree disguised itself as a promotional claim, as a form of national rebranding, as the new public moral standard. The subtle irony of using, in the very name of anti-virus legislation, the hash symbol (#)—a metadata tag endowed with the performative power of making content go *viral* on social networks—went unnoticed in what seemed a confused blur of domains and voices—the voice of state and of the individual voices it addressed (be they citizens, permanent residents, or undocumented migrants) were supposed to come together in a chorus of digital tweets and re-tweets: #IStayHome. The voice of executive power was now speaking in the new register of digital marketing practices. The hashtag now appeared also on my phone's display, next to my provider's name. On the top left corner of the screen a new claim had been juxtaposed to the company's name: Vodafone #IoRestoaCasa. The strategy was successful: the title of the decree became a trendy hashtag.

On March 22, 2020, as midnight was approaching, Premier Giuseppe Conte launched a live video message on his Facebook account to announce a further turn of the screw in the restrictive measures, including the shutdown of all factories producing non-essential goods and drastic limitations in mobility. Public parks were closed and the maximum radius for outdoor walks was set at 200 meters from one's home address.[18] You cannot "travel," stated the decree, "by public or private transport, to a region other than the one in which you are currently located, except for proven work reasons, absolute urgency, or for health reasons." Any outing had to be reported in a self-certification form. Anyone breaking the quarantine rules could be fined and incarcerated. A proliferation of newspapers headlines offered tragicomic stories of people caught in the attempt of gaming the system and ending up being heavily sanctioned: "His hair looked too neat: Stopped by the police, heavy fines for both the customer and the hairdresser"[19]; "Wife hidden in the trunk: they were headed to the beach house"[20]; "Gone for a walk with a sheep on a leash: man fined in Palermo."[21]

New banners stating: "this program has been recorded before the current health emergency," or "this show has been produced before the Decree Law on Coronavirus" had to be mandatorily superimposed on TV programs representing scenes of everyday life from the times before the pandemic, when social distancing norms were not enforced. Virus-related legislation sneaked into our most private sphere, shattering the illusion that there could be a space outside of the disciplinary practices of the state apparatus. The bundles of painstakingly fastidious rules contained in the myriad of executive orders issued in a fast-paced succession for over 8 weeks have grown into a second skin, becoming ingrained into our plague-infested ordinary lives. As the most trivial affairs have become a matter of life or death, executive legislation took charge of our lives, exposing with unprecedented clarity how power is at work even, as Elizabeth Povinelli puts it, "when we seem to be doing nothing more than kissing our lovers goodbye as we leave for the day."[22]

Unexpectedly, and somehow paradoxically, the gradual loosening of the restrictions did not taste like liberation. To the contrary, the country's transition from Phase 1 to Phase 2 reiterated a sense of constriction: now you may walk beyond the vicinity of your homes, walk your dog, or go jogging, maintaining an interpersonal space of at least two meters, or one meter if walking, but you will still be required to carry a self-certification justifying your reason for being outside; while no group gatherings of any kind are allowed, and travel remains strictly limited. A new "reason" was introduced in the narrow list of legitimate purposes for leaving one's home: you may visit your "*congiunti*."[23] The term sounded archaic and opaque to many: does it include non-cohabiting significant others and friends, or does it only refer to relatives ("*parenti*")? And if so, is it just consanguineal relatives or also in-laws? A debate ensued.[24] The semantic scope of the term was later clarified by the Prime Minister: the term "congiunti" applies to spouses, same-sex partners in civil unions, couples who had moved in together but found themselves separated by the lockdown, parents, children, in-laws, siblings, aunts and uncles, nieces and nephews, cousins and cousins' children, who can now be encountered provided the visit complies with the social distancing rules (a one-meter distance, no group gathering, face masks to be used at all times) and does not require traveling inter-regionally. But what about people who are not married and do not live together but are in some form of sexual and sentimental relation? The Prime Minister explained that only those people tied by relations of steady affection would qualify as "congiunti." But how could a police officer determine whether the person you intend to visit actually falls within that category? And what about friends? "No, friends do not qualify as stable affections," specified a note by the government.

Another friend texts me proposing an ingenious plan: perhaps we could meet at the park (now open) wearing face-coverings and pretending to have met by chance? The message amuses me.[25] My friend is smart and knows how to find workarounds exploiting the few liberties that have been restored: parks have been reopened and we are now able to go for longer walks and runs beyond the 200-meter radius from home. But, I think to myself, she is not factoring in that we are still expected to maintain a safe distance from others at all times. A sense of fatigue is upon me. Perhaps I am not as creatively subversive as my friend is, or perhaps I am just too depleted by weeks spent micro-calculating what I can or cannot do. Or perhaps I have just become a prisoner of my own cocoon. I text my friend back saying I am not in the mood to go out. She timidly tries to convince me, but I refuse. I realize I am still incapable of shaking off my new lockdown skin.

Aurora Donzelli

The Other World, or Cacophony and Ethnography in Malaysia

At the time of writing, we *would* have been in Georgetown, Pulau Pinang, in the last week of a summer study abroad fieldwork class training a small group of college students on ethnographic research and writing. Over the past five years, Penang has become sort of a second home for me—a place I would think and pine for during moments of solitude and reflection. I've never lived there for any extended period of time, just a few weeks now and then when I'm on fieldwork or vacation. Something about the island and the city of Georgetown has always felt like home, more so than the city that I grew up in, Kuala Lumpur. This was the summer when we would have brought our baby daughter to visit Malaysia for the first time ever since she was born last October. It had meant to be a trip where she got to meet the other side of her identity—the Southeast Asian one—with all of its many bizarre peculiarities, oddities, and cosmopolitanism.

Not being able to travel back home, especially with our daughter, really hurt, though it's something I don't speak much about. I tell myself that it's just a temporary delay, that at some point in the coming months we will be able to travel again, and that Malaysia (and Penang) will be there waiting for us. It'll have to do.

Penang is a large island of the west coast of Peninsular Malaysia, with a capital city that was a former colonial port town called Georgetown. Back in those days under British imperial rule, the island became an important hub for trade and mercantilism, as well as colonial governance under Francis Light, the British trader and trafficker who is (very problematically) recognized as the founder and first governor of Georgetown. He also happened to be a brutal colonist and slave-owner. A statue of Francis Light on the island was vandalized and smeared with red paint this week in a move that has been tied to the Black Lives Matter movement—though, provincial as ever, the authorities have chosen to simply deem the act as random vandalism.

Penang's subaltern history is fascinatingly complex. The island is home to some of the oldest Chinese migrant settlements in Malaya,[26] a history that has been beautifully preserved in the various clan *kongsi* houses in the oldest parts of the city. It's also home to what used to be the most vibrant and important local fishing communities in the West Coast—many of which include floating villages that one can see while crossing over from the mainland to the island. These days, the island has become home to incredibly diverse groups of people, mostly migrants from neighboring countries and refugees from Burma, living in the same townships as older immigrant communities from India and China.

It would have been the second time that I taught a fieldwork course in Malaysia. Last year's version was one of the best teaching experiences I've ever had, one that was nearly perfectly aligned with my own research and writing, and with students who were so deeply engaged and curious that motivation and inspiration were never in short supply. The premise of the course was simple—teaching students how to conduct ethnographic fieldwork and writing, using displacement, precarity and informality as themes to explore in the everyday life of the city. But that was just the surface of the class—I had a deeper objective to the teaching, which was to get the students to explore and reflect upon a very personal experience of being in "cacophonous" cosmopolitan spaces. The ones where we don't really get to choose or be picky about who, what and how we interact and live with on a daily basis.

The purpose of the lesson was to let students experience difference and diversity in a discomforting and displaced way. Diversity and difference not as a choice based on inclusivity and solidarity, but on necessity and acceptance. Ideas of difference and diversity, in addition to motifs of respect, understanding and alliance, also have to include motifs of hate, prejudice, and bigotry. What happens when diversity and difference are not cherry-picked, selectively included but aspects of daily life that you are forced to encounter and engage each time you step out of your home. I remember the first time explaining this to the students, and getting some very quizzical looks from many, though a couple understood immediately what I meant.

A discordant and cluttered cacophony, rather than a harmonious coming together. Waking up to the sound of the morning call to prayer from a local *surau*, being hit by the smell of strong incense from the neighbors' prayer altar, along with a whole host of smells of food people would already be cooking in homes, from roti to *nasi lemak* to roast pork wontons. There are very few rules about communal behavior among such different and diverse people, but the most important and unspoken one has always been that of tolerance. Not necessarily acceptance or inclusion—invisible boundaries and prejudices abound in everyday life—but above all, you have no choice but to tolerate the everyday cacophony. Trying to fight it, trying to complain, will make one look very foolish indeed. Of course, your neighbors and their families will be up at 5 am and making a racket, of course the local temples, mosques, churches and *tokongs* will be up and ringing their bells and calls to prayer as loudly as possible in an attempt to drown each other out. At an individual level, it can become a trial of learning to accept how little control one can have over one's immediate environment—that closing your doors, building fences, and keeping things out aren't really an option.

Georgetown, Penang, has always been a wonderful case study of this cacophonous urbanity of diversity and difference. It's why I've always felt it would be a perfect place to learn about urban social life, beyond the homogenous and homogenizing tendencies of urbanity in the West. I wanted the group of students—all of whom espouse relatively similar values of acceptance, solidarity and inclusivity couched in love and respect for those who might be different—to experience another type of cosmopolitanism and inclusivity, where prejudice and hate are also possible as part of diversity. A complicated lesson, one that I still have a lot of work trying to improve in terms of how to teach and explain it. I had been excited to try out some new approaches to this, over this summer, but the pandemic put an end to the summer program.

In any case, I'm writing about the cacophony of Penang as a way to work through a strange reality of life in American cities, at least the ones I've been in—Yonkers, New York, Chicago, and Champaign. I grew up used to those cacophonous social life worlds of urban Malaysia, so much so that I never thought about it until they were no longer there. Coming to the United States, especially to the Midwest, I remember being immediately struck by the lack of such cacophony. I was struck by the *tidiness* of it all, how things all fit into perfect little squares and boxes, and how everyday life was governed by so many rules and norms, spoken and unspoken. There were so many expectations and boundaries that one is supposed to respect here, but of course, they almost always favor the orderly, the quiet and the *civilized*. Sounds, loud noises, and cacophonies were *allowed*, only on very specific and special occasions, but one simply does not disturb the neighbors with the sounds of prayer, bells, or even children crying on a daily basis.

It's the lack of the sights, sounds, and smells of religious life that startles me the most in the cities here. In some ways, this is what feels most oppressive, that the only built spaces of worship that are *obvious* are churches, and there simply is no tolerance whatsoever for any sounds of different spiritual lives. No sounds of Islamic calls to prayer, no burning of incense, no chiming of bells from a temple… despite there being different spaces of worship in these cities, they are all built to look fairly similar, or housed within pre-existing buildings that weren't built as places of worship. After a while, it dawned on me that this absence of cacophony likely goes a long way to making these different communities feel very much on the fringes, like they are nothing more than after-thoughts in somebody else's space. *You are more than welcome to practice your spirituality and religion, but make sure it's private or kept within your own communities. The rest of us simply don't want our fragile senses to be bothered by it on a daily basis.*

This different type of urbanity—a powerfully oppressive one—hit me hardest during a trip to Paris in March 2019, where the architecture of the city could not be more antithetical to the kinds of cacophonous diversity I've been describing.

As we spend this summer of the pandemic in the city of Champaign, Illinois, it feels quieter than ever. The only sounds we hear tend to be those we hear within our house, and sometimes the sound of cars and other vehicles passing by. We don't even hear the sounds of children playing outside that much. We don't really hear neighbors being loud. The quiet is sometimes a blessing, when we go for a stroll with the baby around the neighborhood, but increasingly it has become a silence of mourning. We all have our ideal little bubbles here, quaint, cosy, and perfectly sufficient. There's no need to deal with or tolerate any unwanted and unpleasant things from the outside…

Parthiban Muniandy

Communicating with and Through a Face Mask

"Wearing a mask is dangerous."
"You should not wear a mask."
"If you touch the mask in the wrong way, you'll spread the virus on your face. You'll actually get the virus."
"Masks are not appropriate for non-hospital staff."
"Just avoid using masks."

The masks were given to me by a former relative because I am allergic to dust especially during my many moves. I found them in one of my unopened boxes. I was looking for them for days and days. One of my colleagues offered me one of her masks. I refused it. I knew she might need it. Nowhere, were there masks. I knew I had three masks somewhere. I finally found them. Blessed masks. I felt safe.

It was March 2020 and it seemed everyone was against the use of masks. We were very confused about the (non)use of masks, even though we had spare ones, face masks that have traveled with us for a longtime, like my three light blue surgical masks.

My first trip to the supermarket with a mask on was traumatic. I couldn't breathe well. It was not the right mask. I also had to wear gloves to avoid the virus which could linger on charts, groceries, self-checkout touch screens, credit card readers, everywhere… including the surrounding air. Everyone was staring at me, at my light blue surgical mask.

"Why is she wearing a mask? She is not supposed to," I imagined how and what they were thinking by the way they were staring at me. I was terrified.

In Italy, in March, they already asked everyone to wear masks in supermarkets and in other public spaces. They started to distribute masks at supermarkets there when I started to use mine in the US. I purchased a dozen masks on Amazon, just to be safe, even though nobody was using a mask around me yet. I knew that there was a shortage of masks. The masks I ordered arrived two months later. They came from China.

May 11, 2020

Now face masks or face coverings are required in every supermarket and other closed or crowded spaces in New York State. From being scared of wearing masks in March, now people have to wear them and these face coverings have become more visible in closed spaces. There are face masks of various kinds, fabric, color, shape, fantasy, it has become a huge business. New companies are selling masks. In Italy, Gucci prepared masks for everyone two months ago. They are proud of that. A new morality has emerged: We should all use masks because we need to protect others, not ourselves. It is an act of generosity that is not always reciprocated unless it is required such as in supermarkets. Wearing masks has become a political statement.

I wear my face mask all the time when I exit my apartment. Not everyone does so. They are more relaxed, perhaps, they feel they won't need to use the mask, they are young and healthy. Why should they if they don't care? I am terrified of young people not wearing masks and making fun of those who do.

People wearing masks seem to be more silent; they don't seem to be interested in engaging in any kind of communication. It is just awkward. I always try to talk to Marc, one of the maintenance individuals of the complex where I live, when I go out to take my garbage or to take a walk. He used to be very friendly with me. Since I wear my mask diligently, he looks at me as if afraid and avoids eye contact with me. He is silent. Is he scared because I wear a mask? Does he think I am sick? Why has he become so silent? I usually take long walks in the neighborhoods. I am very lucky since I live in a very green, residential area, near the campus where I work. Our campus is closed now, it is almost deserted. It just has some COVID-19 testing stations. What a different picture of a campus that has always been vivacious and full of students. It is completely empty now.

I wear my face mask even when I walk by myself with very few people around me. The other day, during one of these walks, I noted that someone left their beautiful, cloth mask on the ground (Fig. 1.8). Did they throw it away on purpose? Did they do so because they couldn't breathe well? I am tempted to pick it up and to look for the person who has perhaps dropped it. But how can someone accidentally drop a cloth mask like this one? It's there, next to Saint Vincent statue, on the ground, next to a bench where I sit and read when the weather is pleasant.

July 17, 2020

The alarm clock didn't have the time to go off this morning. My phone received tons of messages very early. I woke up to see who was writing to me constantly. A myriad of messages from my family were there to wish me "Happy Birthday." I was supposed to be in Italy this year, as I usually go to celebrate my birthday with my family. The coronavirus is keeping us very united and separate at the same time: united because we are all experiencing similar fears, rules, frustrations, anger; separate, because traveling has become too difficult at the moment, especially when it comes to crossing the Ocean. It will be another day in isolation punctuated by phone calls, birthday wishes, and work.

I decide to take a long walk in search of chipmunks, tiny rabbits, or deer. There are tons of animals out there during this time of the year. I enjoy this area very much. It is my birthday, I should enjoy what I love most: nature. I can also remove my mask when I walk alone. I feel comfortable doing so. I can put it on again when people walk or jog by. They don't seem to pay attention to wearing versus not wearing a mask. They seem to be comfortable with not wearing it. I can't be close to a human being without wearing my mask.

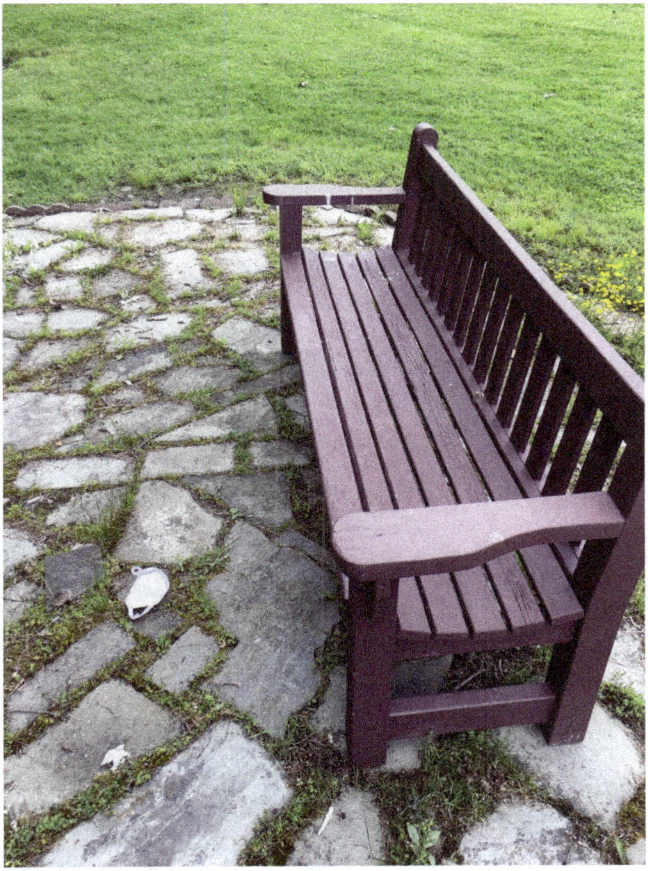

Fig. 1.8 Cloth face mask on the ground. Vestal, New York. May 2020. (Photo by S. M. Perrino)

When I return to my apartment, the mail has already been delivered. I carefully open my mailbox and a bulky envelope from Italy is there. I suddenly remember that my father asked his tailor to make some cloth face masks for me and he said he sent them a month ago. I am sure that this envelope has the tailor-made cloth face masks in it. I get terribly excited. I open the door of my apartment and drop the bulky envelope on the floor. I can't just open it. I need to wait. It is my birthday gift. I need to call my dad first. It is late in Italy, but I call my father anyway. He is so excited about the news of the arrival of his envelope in Vestal. He was hopeless, he confessed.

"With this virus, envelopes can disappear, mail is so delayed, you never know," he says.

"You are right, but the envelope is here now and I'll open it with you on WhatsApp!"

We are both so happy. He, however, is much more excited than I am:

"Do you like them? Nobody will have similar masks in the United States" (Fig. 1.9).

Sabina M. Perrino

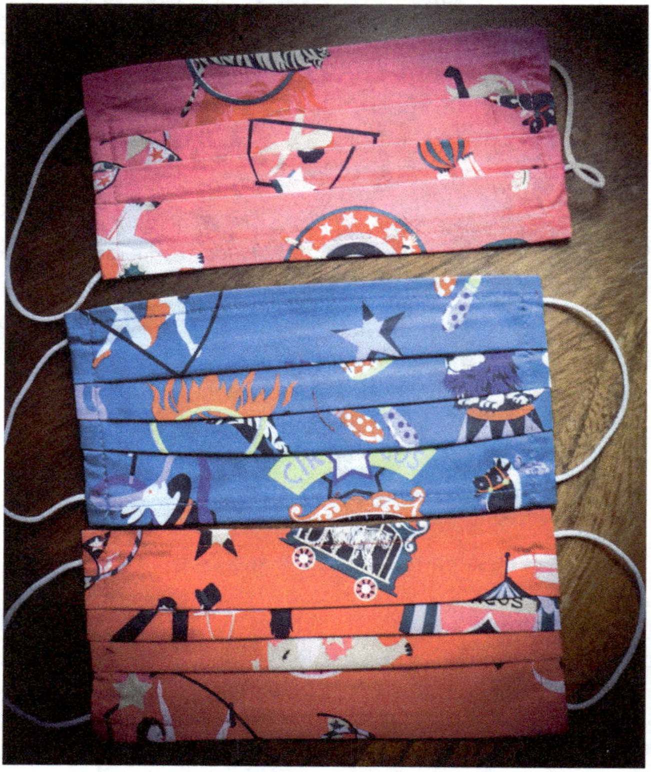

Fig. 1.9 Three Italian, tailor-made face masks. Vestal, New York, July 17, 2020. (Photo by S. M. Perrino)

Family

They aren't wearing masks, they aren't maintaining distance. It is not a political statement, it's a habit borne of hundreds of family gatherings over decades.

I had called a week or two before to establish ground rules for my nephew's graduation party. My parents assumed I called to complain about the presence of his mother (my alcohol-, opiate-, drama-addicted oldest sister). In their defense, I was one of the ringleaders of an improvised intervention two Thanksgivings ago. But that had nothing to do with my call. They then assumed that I wanted to know more about the house in east Rochester that they were renting for the weekend. This was one of many pit stops as they engaged in their annual summer road trip driving from their home in Florida to grandkids and great-grandkids dispersed throughout the Mid-Atlantic and Northeast. They seemed undeterred by the fact that they were heading hundreds of miles in the direction of what had been the epicenter of the global Pandemic. Still trying to guess at the reason for my call, and not yet letting me chime in, the other possibility they offered up was that I wanted to make sure I would get a bed. Of course not, my other older sister (the one with no interest in causing drama) was coming with her husband and two daughters from Pittsburgh to see our nephew and they were occupying one of the rooms. "The couch is fine," I assured them, but my parents were insistent, "you can have a bed, a room…" No, I was finally able to explain, what I really wanted to know when I called was if we were going to abide by social distancing guidelines and not engage in any of the normal intimacy, standing and sitting shoulder to shoulder, hugging, kissing, shaking hands. I was told that we would all be respectful of that and touch elbows instead. I said that is what I wanted.

That is not what they or I did. That is not what happened and I no longer know what I wanted. When I arrived on Friday afternoon, it was just my parents and me. We hadn't seen each other in over six months, though we'd talked on the phone a lot in that time. Every time I called I expected them to say that one of them was sick, but they never were. We hesitated for a moment, then hugged one another. First my dad, then my mom. That night my sister, her husband and two daughters arrived from Pittsburgh. We did the same. The next day I stood around watching the small house fill up, my sisters and their daughters, the significant others for my eldest two nieces, my brother and his girlfriend, our other nephew and his girlfriend, my mother's youngest sister and her husband, me, my nephew and my parents. Four parts of New York state were represented, Utica, Auburn, Rochester and Binghamton. Florida and Pittsburgh were there. There were more hugs, more handshakes and close talking. And when it was over we all went back to where we came from.

I hugged and shook hands and stood close to people who weren't my wife and son for the first time in months. It felt good. Maybe because epidemics are just as abstract as geographic distance, but family feels more real. Maybe because it was the first trip I had taken in months, after campus visits, conferences, travel for my wife and I were canceled, one event after another. Maybe because it was the first night in a long time that I had had away from somewhat taxing childcare responsibilities with our disabled son. Maybe it was just the exhilarating thought of being close to people I loved other than my wife and child, sharing stories and breaking bread with them. I hugged and I shook hands.

My parents have just arrived in Florida, a week later, after visiting more friends in New York and Pennsylvania, and relatives in North Carolina and the D.C. area. I'll wait another week, enough time for the virus to manifest in symptoms as far as I know, to see if we all made a terrible mistake. In a month we might call them carriers, we might worry for their health or ours. In a month, all that intimacy and shared memory might develop a menacing tone in our collective imaginations. Or not. Maybe death for some or all, maybe nothing. The virtuality of pandemic, the virtuality of family. Both so intimate.

Josh Reno

Sanitizing New York

I felt reassured, even proud.

Though I hadn't generally followed Governor Andrew Cuomo's daily briefings, I did happen to catch a snippet of his March 9th address. New York State, Cuomo announced, was producing its own brand of hand sanitizer—NYS Clean. I spent less than a minute absorbing the news, but remember feeling the positive boost it had on my mood. Later happenings cause me to return to the archived recording of this press conference that would have otherwise faded into the background hum of constant updates about the pandemic to ask: What had I found to be so comforting about Cuomo's message? (Fig. 1.10).

The appeal of this particular news conference derived in part from its positioning as a response to recent failures in the national government leadership and private markets. The launch occurred at a time when

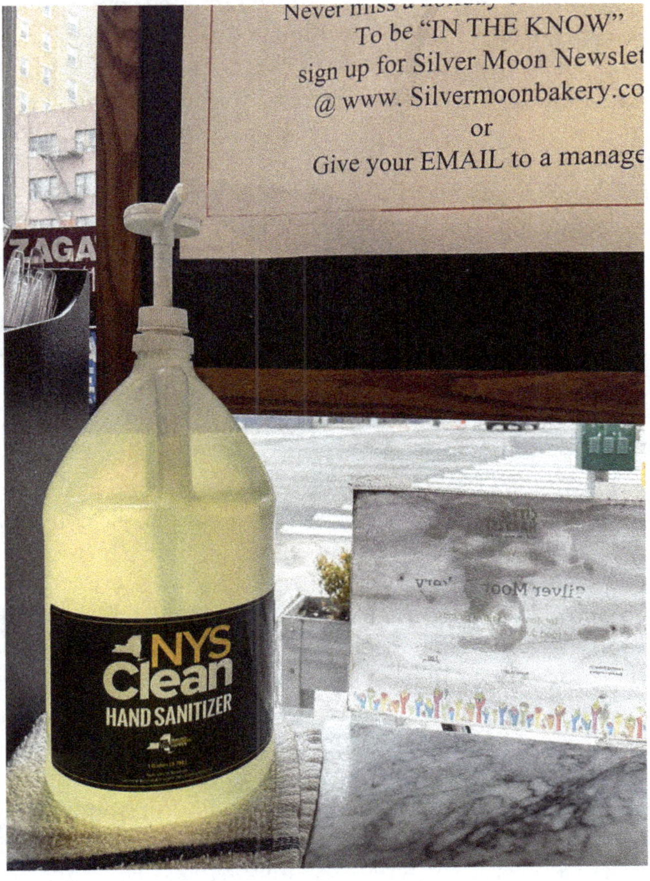

Fig. 1.10 NYS Clean Hand Sanitizer. (Photo by J. Jacobs)

widespread shortages of PPE, ventilators, toilet paper, and other essentials co-existed with reports of predatory online vending practices and a grim realization of the costs of diminished domestic production of many health-related commodities. Standing in front of hundreds of bottles of NYS Clean, Cuomo noted that the state sanitizer was not only a "good deal," produced at the bargain price of just over six dollars a gallon, but that, with its alcohol content in line with WHO guidelines and pleasing scent, was a superior product to Purell. The semiotics of the simple green and white NYS Clean letters on a black background conveyed local rather than foreign, public instead of private, and enlightened straight-talking, action-oriented democratic leadership compared to the obstructionist, mendacious messaging offered in Trump's competing daily COVID briefings.

NYS Clean sanitizer also referenced a new solidarity forged between New Yorkers under siege. The hand sanitizer was made by "ourselves, not on the open market" and distributed to "us." The governor's boldly asserted "we" appeared to unify producers and consumers, government employees and citizens, in the circulation of a potentially life-saving commodity as an act of solidarity. This was one small part of a broader effort of New Yorkers to care for each other in a time of crisis.[27]

A couple weeks after the press conference, the arrival of a letter marked the beginning of my own far more complicated feelings about NYS Clean. I first met its author, Juan, the previous year while working as a volunteer at the Parole Preparation Project (PPP), an abolitionist organization dedicated to helping people with life sentences advocate for their release from state confinement. He offered a brief update on life in Great Meadow, a maximum-security state prison north of Albany. While college courses and other activities in the prison had been put on hold, the recently converted "soap shop" now operated 24 hours a day. Workers in three shifts paid a fraction of the state's minimum wage ensured the delivery of 100,000 gallons of NYS Clean sanitizer a week. Production was overseen by Corcraft, the public face of the New York State Department of Corrections and Community Supervision's Division of Industries.

The letter also documented the impact of the prison's woefully inadequate response to COVID-19. Testing at the time was not available to people who were detained, guards and medical personnel were often not wearing masks, and social distancing while moving through the indoor spaces—especially the cafeteria—was impossible. Juan noted he was "afraid every time inmates are coughing in the hallway and everywhere." NYS

Clean sanitizer was considered contraband if it left the soap shop—incarcerated people only had access to handkerchiefs and soap, which they were unable to use while moving around the prison.

Juan's descriptions evoked my own memory from a previous trip to the prison where I had walked past a group of ten men, most of whom were Black, stripping paint from the steps, supervised by two white guards in this facility sitting on farmland in an overwhelmingly white part of the state. The particularly stark visceral embodiment of racial capitalism was now connected to the life-saving hand sanitizer emblazoned with the state brand.

It is July. Releasing Aging People in Prison (RAPP) recently organized a rally in the state capital to commemorate the lives of 48 incarcerated people who died of COVID while in state custody. After state parole board members denied his parole in February, Juan also recently heard that his application for emergency COVID release due to a preexisting condition had been rejected.

My partner and I have been trying to arrange a visit to see Juan. Prison officials initially mistakenly tell us that state pandemic rules kept them from granting us an appointment. After finally receiving approval from the authorities, concerned family members tell me the planned visit is an "extreme" thing to do in the midst of the pandemic. I relent and we schedule a legal phone call with Juan instead of the in-person visit. It is awkward conversation, filled with long silences. He hates the phone. I feel frustrated that the visit didn't happen, and guilty that I wasn't able to spend even a few hours visiting in the prison where he had been staying for more than a decade.

NYS Clean is still being distributed widely throughout the state. I recently saw a large bottle prominently displayed on the table at an outdoor bar. I had a brief urge to grab it—I'm not exactly sure for what purpose. Instead, I purchased a bottle of hand sanitizer at the local pharmacy. As Purell and other familiar names were unavailable, I picked up a bottle called M Skincare. I had never spent much time thinking about hand sanitizers, but now, I notice the cool slippery sensation as it spreads over my hands and the amount of time it takes to dry and sniff my fingers to see if has left a distinctive smell. The label on the bottle tells me the product was "designed and developed in the U.S.A, manufactured in China." Suddenly, I find myself wondering if it was made in detention centers employing compulsory labor; Uighurs or perhaps even people with heroin use history who I came to know during my previous fieldwork in China might have helped to make this product in miserable conditions. Of course, these are just my associations. There is no immediate way for me to find out.

As I finish writing this dispatch, an internet search turns up a new, unsettling piece of information. NYS Clean, as it turns out, is *bottled* at Great Meadow and two other prison facilities. However, the sanitizing liquid arrives at the prisons from somewhere else—a "mysterious vendor" that the state refuses to identify.[28] Cuomo's "we," as it turns out, could include workers from anywhere, but what care have they been offered? I find myself returning to the dirty promises behind clean hands.

Nicholas Bartlett

On Shopping and the Desire to Buy Shit During a Pandemic

We weren't sure what to expect, but it was never going to be this. Bustling throngs of people. Interspersed by long lines on the pavement of people queuing due to social distancing requirements, all along the sidewalks of the outdoor mall in Yonkers, New York. It was only days after New York entered Phase 3 of the reopening, which allowed for most businesses, including retail, to be open to customers. Of the things that we would have been desperate to do once being able to go outside again, shopping seems like an odd choice—especially shopping in large crowded malls.

But there we were, staying in a hotel right in the middle of a crowded mall, where most people weren't even bothering with face masks, and families with children were happily milling about from store to store, playground to playground, in what felt like a mockery of the pandemic we're living under. There were warnings and advisories posted all over, on the sidewalks, on the walls, doors, and entrances, telling everyone to wear a mask and practice distancing. It's amazing how quickly these things become white noise to us—just like any other sign or advert that we tune out for convenience.

This was the fourth day of our drive from Illinois to New York, an unexpected trip that we had to make to move some of our things out of the apartment in Yonkers. The drive itself had been incredibly, surreally, smooth, and uninterrupted. Despite the lockdowns, shelter-in-place and travel restrictions that were in place in various states, there were no visible signs of any sort of enforcement on the road. The pinnacle of surrealness was at the point we got on to the George Washington Bridge into Manhattan, and were able to drive through to the city at 11.30 am with minimal traffic *on a Tuesday.* We had been expecting roadblocks and checks upon entering the different states—Indiana, Ohio, West Virginia, Pennsylvania, New Jersey, and New York—in some form or another, but the only block we found was a road closure due to a minor landslide somewhere along the Pennsylvania turnpike. I suppose COVID-19 doesn't really bother with roads and highways, since air travel and cruise ships seem to be all the rage.

One part of me is baffled by the almost desperate desire people seem to have with shopping and buying stuff, even during a severe and unprecedented public health crisis, with a virus that spreads so quickly and widely. What is it that drives us to feel we need to buy *stuff* so badly, that we are willing to risk going out to crowded spaces—old and young, of all races and genders—and line up to enter stores? Could it be that retail therapy is far more effective than we realized? Could it be that under such conditions of a pandemic, shopping malls and retail outlets become one of the only possible ways we are able to see other people and socialize in some form? Or could it be that such is the state of our contemporary social life that the only way we can express our existence and presence during a pandemic is through our wallets and our capacity to purchase things we don't need?

It's hard for me not to feel a bit annoyed and judgmental of those who crowd these shopping malls (especially as we were carrying an infant with us and desperately trying to keep her away from the crowds), but something else tempers this feeling. My own inclinations and urges to want to leave and go outside, especially as a parent of an infant dealing with a lockdown, often translates into random and frequent compulsions to look at things I could *buy.* Mostly, this manifests in browsing Amazon, Best Buy, or Newegg, to look for things on sale that I could use to build computers, as a way of dealing with the boredom of occupying an infant who has just learned to crawl in the middle of the day. (I've been a technophile since my days as a teenaged electronics pirate/thief/black market vendor in Malaysia). Sometimes, the boredom and desire to do *something* threatens to be overwhelming, and I'd feel desperate to pack the baby in her car seat and drive to the local IT store, or a café with a drive-thru, or somewhere I can just do *anything*, and that *anything* inevitably ends up spending some money to buy *something.*

It feels like a bizarre and twisted form of agency during COVID times, a way for us to enact some action we feel is silently defiant, against a larger institutional force we really can't do much against except comply. I really just want to be able to buy a ticket and fly back to Malaysia with my baby daughter, to have her meet her grandparents and friends there, to take her to my favorite island towns in Penang and Langkawi, to have her experience the heat and humidity of the former rubber plantations where one half of her ancestors are from, to sit with her by the roadside hawker stalls on Gurney Drive where I wrote so many of my books and essays in the past decade… but I can't buy that ticket, so instead I'm going to give COVID-19 the middle finger and go buy myself a white chocolate mocha and that utterly unnecessary but shiny new solid state drive from Best Buy. What might we call this—defiance of the consumer? Wallet agency? Credit-card resistance? In corona times, can the consumer speak?

Jokes aside, what it really feels like is funereal. Bodies and people milling and shuffling about desperately longing for a bygone time, in spaces that are little more than ghost towns now. Highly sanitized, over-policed ghost towns, but ghost towns nonetheless. Retail outlets and shopping malls like the one we came across seem more and more like those old cowboy towns in Southeast Asia that used to be thriving economic hotbeds but have long since been left behind by urbanization and modern development, yet spaces where people are still desperate to recover and reenact what used to be.

So, in one way, I do understand that urge to shop and buy stuff, at least from this perspective. I don't quite get how strong the desperation could be to be willing to get into crowds, however.

Parthiban Muniandy

The Workout

It is Saturday morning and my alarm clock has just reminded me of my upcoming class at my local gym: bootcamp with Sophia at 8:30am. I rush to the bathroom to brush my teeth, while preparing my nutritious breakfast that I will be able to eat after the workout. I can't really eat before exercising with Sophia. Any kind of food would make me feel nauseous after the first five minutes of her intense workout. But I have some water with electrolytes in it just in case I need it. I need to rush. I just put on some gym clothes very quickly. It is freezing cold outside but my car will be warm soon. I race through the empty highway. It's only 7:45a.m. I have plenty of time. Yet, I know that Sophia will be there to set up the room at 7:50am. For some reason, I am always there to help her and to chat with her. That's the only time I can chat with Sophia. It has become a ritual. I just can't miss bootcamp. This time I will wear a mask, however, which is something new for me and for all the participants. I am just very curious to see how class goes with everyone wearing a mask. Will we be able to do the usual strenuous workouts that Sophia proposes?

I park my car at the gym and I see Sophia's car already parked there. It makes me feel good to see her car. I feel as if I were at home again. I knew I was a bit late than usual. I feel terribly tired, however, my eyes are heavy, but I just want to be there. I take all my things in my locker and get ready for crossing the common gym space to get to the studio where classes are usually taught. While I walk through the gym, I note that gym members do not wear their face masks. I am a bit confused about the new rules of my gym. Hopefully, I will be able to exercise with my face mask on.

"Good morning, Sabina," says Sophia as soon as she sees me. Her eyes are sparkling.

"We need to set all the benches in two or three rows, one close to the other one," she says to me.

She talks as if we have seen each other in person every single Saturday morning, which was definitely the case before this pandemic. I haven't seen her face-to-face in three months. It has been a long time. Why is she so cold with me? I want to hug her and show her that I am smiling of happiness. My face mask is blocking the view of my lips. All of a sudden, I note that she is not wearing a mask. I am too tired to start asking questions and the only thing I want to do is to hug her, which I can't do since I need to keep my distance from her. Why is she behaving so "normally"? I wish I could do so too.

"OK, Sophia, I'll do so," I say enthusiastically. "I'll start from here to build the first row of benches."

I like building the first row, the one that reflects my image in the mirror. I like to build every bench precisely before adding the equipment that we need. I select my bench, next to Sophia's, as always. I can't be too far from her. The workout is so intense and fast that I need to see what she does and how the new moves take shape from her experienced body. I am always so scared to fall from the bench while jumping up and down and to hurt myself. Why do I do this? It is so early, I shouldn't even think too much about this and just do it.

"Do we need the barbell or only dumbbells?" I ask her once all the twenty-two benches are perfectly aligned in three long rows.

“Barbell and dumbbells, Sabina, you know it, and kettlebells too,” says Sophia while walking fast from one end to the other end of the room while adding long, red rubber bands to every bench.

“Of course, I know it, I just wanted to make sure,” I say while smiling at her, although she can’t see my lips because they are covered by my face mask. Perhaps, she can see that I smile at her because my eyes might have a different shape when I smile or laugh. She seems to be in a very good mood. She always is before teaching her bootcamp class.

She doesn’t even question my use of the mask. Did she actually see that I am using my face mask? She needs to use one too. This is one of the many new rules to be able to take classes in gyms in New York State! Or… is it not?

I start building my own barbell first with the weights that are good for me. I am so weak, I don’t feel like lifting heavy weights today. I just can’t in the morning. Sophia knows my rituals, she knows my body. She has observed me while struggling with the exercises that she proposes. I feel as if she knows every muscle of my body, she has scrutinized me while I practice, she has performed X-rays with her attentive eyes. I am not hiding my many weaknesses from her. And, yet, participants are so competitive in her classes. She always challenges me and she will challenge me today as well.

I am alone in the room for a moment. I take a break. I sit on my bench, I stretch my legs. I look at myself in the mirror: I can just see my eyes, my face mask is covering my face, my mouth, my nose. Will I be able to exercise with this face covering on me? Sophia is in the bathroom. She is still not wearing her face mask when she comes back. I am a bit surprised and feel anxious about this. Her reassuring smile catches me. I wish I could smile back. I am smiling back, but she cannot see it.

It is 8:25am. It’s late, we will start class in 5 minutes. Sophia is very punctual. Late comers are not always welcome. Participants start getting in the room, they take their own bench, they modify their equipment by adding different types of dumbbells, they stretch and chat with Sophia and with each other. The room is almost full. There are already twenty participants. I have people next to me, they are too close to me. What’s going on? Nobody seems to respect the required safe distance of six feet. To my dismay, they are not wearing their masks either. None of them! I am shocked. I am scared. I’ll get infected for sure today. They look at me as if I didn’t have a mask on either. I just don’t want to get infected. I should just leave the room right now. Perhaps, I should say that I am not feeling well, that I need a break, that I can't jump with a mask on. But what if they tell me: "just remove your mask"... would I remove it?

"Let's warm it up guys," says Sophia while starting her fast moves with the loud music accompanying them.

OK, I'll just do the warm-up and I will go away. I love her bootcamp warm-up. It is the same all the time. I can just do it with my eyes completely closed. We now start with the first exercise on the bench.

"Toe taps for one minute or even longer, we'll see," says Sophia while starting her toe tap jumps on her bench.

She can see everyone through the mirror. Her eyes are scrutinizing us. I start jumping up and down my bench. It is really solid, I should not worry. I won't fall. It will be fine. It is just one minute of jumps after all. It is nothing. My mask starts being heavy on my face. Nobody has noted it yet. They don't seem to care. They are all jumping up and down.

My legs hurt. I need to stop. All of a sudden, I feel as if my legs were completely blocked, paralyzed. I am stuck within my pain, I can't move anymore. Sophia will see me soon and she will stop instructing to help me. I am incapable of moving. I am paralyzed in my own body.

I am completely drenched in sweat when I open my eyes at 7:00a.m., just fifteen minutes before my alarm clock goes off. I put my hands on my face to see if I wear a mask. I don't. I am in my bed, it is early morning, why should I wear a mask? I need to wake up, take a shower and get ready for Sophia's Zoom class. Who knows what she'll teach today. She changes all the time. We meet at 8:30a.m. Nobody wears a mask. We all exercise from our own living rooms, kitchens, bedrooms, garages, patios, even offices at workplaces. I will be able to smile back at her today. That makes me feel thoroughly human.

Sabina M. Perrino

No Mask

My wife and I have a small joke we use when driving. When someone passes us by in a hurry, breaking speed limits and driving erratically, one of us says, "they are probably in labor and headed to the hospital." I started it. It sounds like something my sisters or mom would have come up with, so I imagine I heard it from one of them first. Of course, the idea behind this is that you never know what is going on in other people's lives and, therefore, are in no position to judge their actions, however much you might want to. It also centers on an unborn child, which also fits with my family's American heteronormative-liberal-Catholic tendency to place reproduction (and vulnerable children in particular) at the center of all moral reasoning, as if that were the supreme value trumping all others.

After a decade and a half raising our disabled son, Charlie, my wife and I have extended that saying into an all-purpose philosophy.

Someone at the chemical plant where she works asks to take additional time off to be home with their child during the Pandemic. Her co-workers laugh and mock, "His kid's over 18! That's bullshit!" Jeanne responds, "maybe they have a disability and need home care, you don't know."

A person we barely know comes up to us on the street and starts babbling about the gym we all used to work out at being closed. They don't make eye contact or respond to conversational cues. "He might be on the spectrum," I suggest afterward. My wife and I share knowing nods.

Maybe we do this in part because we know how people might misinterpret what they see our son do. We hope strangers will extend him, and us, the same benefit of the doubt. They might think that we are pinching his ear as we walk together because we are leading him angrily out the door, when he put our hand there for the sensory stimulation. They might not understand why he doesn't respond when they say "hello!" or "what's your name?" when he can't speak. They might see him without a mask on.

Today, I got a call from one of our son's daytime caregivers. She had already left for the day and, as it happened, I was playing with Charlie when she called. I wouldn't normally answer the phone, but we always worry when we get unexpected calls from staff, maybe something is wrong or something came up and we will need to rearrange our schedules last minute and Charlie will be affected by the change in plans (people on the spectrum don't normally respond well to breaks in routine). In Charlie's case, he also doesn't respond well when we talk on the phone in front of him, which he really hates. I answer and listen long enough to hear her explain that the reason she is calling is that there was an incident earlier that day she forgot to mention. Someone got aggravated when they saw Charlie get on and off the elevator without a mask on. Charlie normally leaves the apartment once or twice a day with one of us, usually to drive around, sometimes to go to the park. With no school, it is the only opportunity he has for time anywhere but at home. We worry if school remains closed to him, he is going to settle into being a hermit and having little to no social interaction outside of our small circle. And we've never been able to get him to wear a mask (he also won't wear hats, helmets, earplugs, or headphones and resists brushing his teeth, getting his nails clipped or hair cut). In all this time during the Pandemic, no one has ever said anything to us about it when we have been in public, but we always worried they would. Now it's finally happened.

Our carer didn't know whether it was an employee of our apartment building or a resident, but thought we should know. I was bothered by the reported incident, but not as bothered as Charlie was that I'd answered the phone. So much so that I had to tell her to text me the details and then set about calming him down for the next twenty minutes with reassuring words, my phone far out of reach, and deep pressure massages of his fingers and toes. Here is the text that came shortly after, which I read once he calmed down and reprint with permission:

> I'm so sorry to bother you, and it really wasn't that big of a deal but I just wanted to let you know in case it happened again. I couldn't tell if it was someone who worked in the apartment complex or if it was someone who lived there, but he had a few things on a cart to load onto the elevator while we were getting off of it. He was an older guy, he had a mask and a baseball cap on. That was all I could make out of him because I was more concerned about getting Charlie out of the building. When we got off the elevator he said to me once "he is supposed to have a face mask on" and then I just looked at him and continued walking out, and then he again said "it's required. A face mask is required and he needs one" very rudely. I know that people can be very ignorant sometimes that's why I didn't respond to him, but I thought it was something I should tell you.

Here is what I wrote back:

> I spoke with the front office of the building

I had. The manager there also has a disabled child, whom we've never met but who she says is a lot like our son.

> If someone ever mentions that again, you can just say "He's medically exempt from using a mask."

The apartment manager claims she is exempt too, as is her son. She carries around paperwork to that effect and during another incident she did not describe in much detail, she was asked to show another aggrieved person who had noticed she was maskless. She assured us that we did not need to have similar paperwork for our son, not on their building's premises anyway, and we were doing nothing wrong. I wrote our carer back, finally:

> Or you can say nothing, you choice [sic]

I am comforted by the fact that the people who run our apartment complex we live in are supportive of us. On the other hand, I do not know if they would be, if the manager did not happen to have a very similar experience she was living through with her child.

I am also painfully aware that (like the "in labor on the way to the hospital" joke/aphorism that I like to tell while driving) my dispatch is another child-centric account. I do not know what childless people with medical conditions, or with disabilities less obvious, less popularly "sympathetic" than my son's, are going through when they are found maskless or, contrariwise, when they find themselves in a panic in proximity to someone they don't know who is maskless. I do know I had a different reaction to the woman who was widely criticized for refusing to wear a mask at a Starbucks in San Diego weeks ago. After forgetting to bring her medical exemption when she went out, and was denied service, the woman posted an angry and public Facebook message about the barista who would not serve her. The barista then received over $100,000 in go fund me tips as the general public demonstrated with whom, between the two, they'd had sympathy.

I am not overly sympathetic with anyone who turns to social media to garner sympathy or insult people who work in the service industry, to be honest. But I know I thought about doing both those things, possibly, if only for a second, after my son was criticized by a stranger who may or may not have been an employee of the building. And I don't know what my son might face when he's older, less of a child, less of a recognizable "victim" in need of protection, but still sensitive about covering his face when it's expected.

My wife and I have another small joke we like to make when we are out on social occasions and we get bored, or are invited to them and would like to back out. "We can't" (we say, laughing to ourselves and no one else), "his autism is really flaring up." "Sorry, he's having a bad autism… a lot of autism today." This is partly funny to us because it deliberately mis-characterizes autism as if it were an acute medical issue, like a rash or fever. It is also rarely true, but reflects assumptions that well-meaning friends and family make out of ignorance. The fact is, our son can put up with most any situation (as long as we are not on the phone) and routinely surprises everyone with how resilient he is about, for instance, the entire country and his school closing down for several months. I really doubt that the attempt at public shaming earlier today had much of any impact on him at all for that reason. Though I know that I'm going to be thinking about it the rest of the week and will weigh whether or not to tell my wife for the rest of the day. I probably won't, I don't want to worry her. It's not like I tell her about every bad car accident I nearly get into while driving because I imagine someone else is having a baby. And I don't really know the perspective of the person, our possible neighbor, that possible employee. Who knows what they might be dealing with? Maybe they have loved ones that they worry will get sick.

But also, by that same token, fuck them for being rude to my kid.

Josh Reno

Queer life in Quarantine

Mid-April 2020

Even as an out gay man in Chicago before the COVID-19 pandemic, opportunities to be among fellow queers are not easy to come by. Before March 2020, to meet up with my friends at a Northside gay bar, I would have to coordinate via text and take a 45-minute trip by public transit, or I would have to wait for summertime parades, festivals, and marches organized by fellow queers. Looking back upon these experiences, I realized that physical co-presence among gay men is something that could only happen in particular spaces and particular times: one could wear a provocative Speedo to the approval of onlookers only during summertime in Chicago's Hollywood Beach, and one could sing loudly to Madonna tunes only during 80s' nights at a particular gay bar.

In mid-March, however, virtually all of Chicago's vibrant queer nightlife scene was shut down, leaving myself and many other queers to wonder when they will meet each other again. I thought about queers who retreated to their own homes, often by themselves, often without a source of income, and often in places where they cannot safely express their own sexuality. Thus, during the pandemic, I feel as if social distancing policies assume that one's own social life could be confined by the four walls of a building, away from supposed strangers and supposed non-kin. There are those, though, like me, whose sociality are not defined by the walls of a single building: as a gay man, just like other queers, I rely on shared physical spaces outside of my own home to feel that I can be among others who are like me. Before long, however, new forms of queer sociality emerged.

In the first few months of the pandemic, one queer space that emerged is the virtual party, hosted via Zoom, a web conference tool that has become globally ubiquitous. Instead of facilitating a meeting or a seminar, however, Zoom unexpectedly provided a way for friends and strangers alike to recreate queer nightlife spaces online. DJs, drag performers, and other artists would organize these nights with a particular theme, and attendees would participate by clicking a link that is sent through a closed mailing list. Among attendees who have their videos turned on, I often see clothing that I associate with the queer nightlife scene—clothing that would not make it to heteronormative Zoom classrooms or video conference meetings. Rather than a neatly buttoned shirt or a blouse, Zoom party attendees wore leather harnesses that accentuate their physique, tight-fitting tank tops or T-Shirts, or no shirt at all. However, unlike a gay bar or any other nightlife venue for queers, there is simply no possibility of an in-person physical encounter—you can chat through instant messages, and you can invite others to check your social media profiles for more photos and videos, but that is all.

Through these Zoom parties, one avoids the costs and consequences of in-person encounters, even if these risks are not necessarily tied to the COVID-19 pandemic: one can be younger than 21 (the legal drinking age in the US) as long as one is older than 18, one does not need to have enough money for a cab ride home, and one does not have to pay for cover charges and drinks. Furthermore, these Zoom parties do not offer the possibility of in-person sexual encounters—something that is charged with both excitement and anxiety among gay men who are well-aware that sex, life, and death have been deeply intertwined since the AIDS pandemic of the 1980s.

Oddly enough, I felt as if these Zoom parties leveled the playing field for anyone who wishes to enjoy queer nightlife, because, this time around, I was not the only one standing awkwardly at the edge of a dance floor with one or two friends. Everyone, including myself, tried their best to make use of the awkward angles that laptop video cameras provide.

While streaming DJ sets through Twitch, an online streaming platform, I enjoyed scrolling through the video boxes in Zoom that represent individual participants. As I scroll, I saw a multitude of poses that provide a contrast to the uniformity of sitting for Zoom meetings and Zoom classrooms. During these Zoom parties, I saw a person lying down on a couch while nursing a drink, a handful of friends dancing in a dark living room lit by a disco ball, and a couple chatting the night away as they navigate their laptop screen. However, unlike interacting at a gay bar, where I would mostly interact on a one-on-one basis to another person, I had the choice of addressing all party attendees at once by choosing the "message everyone" function.

"Looking good everyone!" I typed, trying to get a positive mood launched as people gradually log-in. A few hours later, just after midnight, I remembered seeing almost 200 attendees, with about a third of them turning their cameras on.

"Happy Beltane boys!!!" someone else typed, referencing a queer May Day tradition of nationwide gatherings that was canceled due to the pandemic.

"Nice harness," said one participant to me as they referred to the leather accessory I wore.

In a blend of anonymity and intimacy that I associate with interactions in queer nightlife settings, I never exchanged names, hometowns, or jobs at these gay nightlife events over Zoom. I simply had the pleasure of knowing that these people have something in common with me.

Late July 2020

A few months later, as the heat of Chicago's scorching summer peaked, I biked along Lake Michigan to investigate what had happened after the closure of Hollywood Beach, Chicago's traditional gathering place for gay men. Much like their predecessors who congregated in Belmont Rocks, a now-disappeared patch of parkland along Lake Michigan, gay men have found other spots along the lakefront to gather with their friends and lovers. A somewhat risky proposition during the COVID-19 pandemic, of course, and yet one that reminds me of a kind of mortality that another generation of queers encountered—death and disease during the AIDS pandemic in the 1980s and early 1990s, before the advent of successful retroviral treatments. Would it be better, I thought, to take risks and live a good life, or to live so fearfully, as if every form of physical intimacy would irretrievably hurt?

I kept biking, by myself, wearing a mask that was increasingly uncomfortable in hot weather. But the 90-degree heat finally got the better of me. I stepped off my bike and walked along the lake's rocky barriers, where I tried my best to maintain physical distance from others who were gathering in groups small and large. Still, I long for the company of queers who share these spaces too. To me, life as a gay man means constantly reinventing kinship, friendship, and companionship by interacting with strangers and new acquaintances. When would I be comfortable hanging out again in a beach that is crowded, shoulder-to-shoulder, with others who, at most, wear a tight-fitting Speedo? When can I enjoy dancing to disco music again with strangers (or, sometimes, newly made friends)? As I sat down on the grass, wiping sweat from my forehead, I said to myself: soon, very soon

Rafadi Hakim

Stroud Playground

I walked by this cement rectangle with its patch of grass, basketball court, and picnic tables nearly every day on my COVID stroll of sanity. Parks and playgrounds have taken on a new meaning in 2020 becoming, for many of us, a central site of collectivity crucial to civic, recreational, and social life.

Mid-April 2020: The cops were in their usual spot. In a deadpan voice, they called out over the loudspeaker: "Don't you know," pausing for effect, "we are living through a pandemic. Get off the playground." The woman with her silky black wig pulled low over her forehead glanced over at the white SUV with the blue stripe running down its middle. Her kids, all under the age of ten, shimmied up and down the slides, and slid their hands along the metal pipes of the jungle gym. I imagined their little hands spreading "corona." The woman tugged at her thick knee-length puffy coat, her long skirt peeking out from underneath. "Off the playground," the cops called out. What would it be like to live through this pandemic in a house full of people?

Mid-July 2020: Kids on bikes, some on trikes. Teens learned to kickflip on skateboards. Gen-Zer's zoomed around on light-up roller-skates flashing red, green, and yellow. Millennial moms power walked. Young men did sit-ups, push-ups, pull ups. All of them circled the boys and girls playing basketball. The players touched, they pushed, they pulled. The steady pulse of the basketball punctuated by the shrill of sneakers rubbing against the pavement. Competing speakers blare U Know What's Up by Donnell Jones, Dead to Me by Kali Uchis, and Wait a Minute! By Willow. Jones' voice carries across the playground: "Oo, say what? Say what? Say what? Yeah. Ooh girl you know, what's up?"

Early August 2020: The hot night wind brought some respite from the heavy, humid days. I sat cross-legged on a bench between Park Place and the basketball court, wearing my summer uniform: short jean overalls, a tank top, and white high-top converse. A curvy woman in long braids danced to her own soundtrack: phone in hand, headphones in ears, hips swaying, to back-to-back salsa tracks. She stepped side to side, front to back, crisscrossing her feet along a line only she could see. She nodded at me, her audience of one.

Mid-August 2020: It was my second to last night in New York. In the fierce heat, the sweet smell of BBQ smoke drifted toward me and my friend. A pudgy cop in glasses and a buzz cut leaned against the railing of the nearly empty playground, watching us get closer. "Even with your masks," he said with a flirtatious tone in a thick Brooklyn accent, "I can *still* see you laughing at my smart car." "Why is there *always* one of *you* here, in this exact spot?" my friend asked. "Because of all the gang activity and drive by shootings," he answered. A subway whistled way off. I can still feel his eyes on our backs as the two of us walked away. We reached the bodega on the corner of Classon and Park, and took deep breaths of the long wet night.

Margaux Fitoussi

Touch (In Progress)

It has been 130 days (I think) since I was touched or touched someone. I used to touch and be touched often. It seemed like nothing to rest a hand on a colleague's arm having tea in the kitchen of our office. I spent most of last November in Argentina and I was scheduled to fly back in March, but flights were canceled and the border is still closed. Something I love about Argentina is the profligacy of touch. When I am there, I take tango classes sometimes for many hours a day, so that involves a lot of touch of course. But even everyday interactions are rich in touch. Hugs last longer, friends will hold your arm more often. Whenever I come back to Europe or the US, I feel lonely for that easy touch and miss it. Perhaps from years of tango, I have saved up some touch, stowed in dromedary fashion and this is what I am surviving on now.

My fieldwork involved working in forensic labs. In my dissertation, I wanted to talk about how, in the apprenticeship of forensics, so much is learned through touch—the texture of fractures that indicates the timing of a wound, the texture of bones that helps determine age. I wanted to explore the qualities of touch that I noticed as people lay their hands on bodies—sometimes clinical, sometimes tender. But I found it very hard to write about touch. I have little vocabulary for describing its quality, or discussing differences in textures. And thus touch—so tangible and material, also proved to be ephemeral.

My failed attempt to write about touch makes me think of how, before film and video, dancers attempted to annotate choreography, scoring movements like notes of music. These notations always struck me as quaint, an attempt both whimsical and doomed. As I look at them now, they seem more urgent, less comedic. The gap between bodies and memory cannot be bridged maybe.

In forensic labs, touch is a skill to be studied and mastered. Some people were better at it than others. Some people could ascertain subtleties in the textures of the bone that my fingertips were numb to. People who are blind develop greater tactile sensitivity in their fingertips because they use their sense of touch more frequently than people with sight.[29] I worry vaguely that I am losing touch. I find it hard to remember touch: what it feels like exactly, precisely. The other day, I watched a YouTube video of a tango dancer I know. We have danced together. I worked carefully to try to place myself into the dance. I tried to feel the exact pressure of his hand on my back. It was difficult to conjure. It was no easy fantasy; it was laborious like conjugating verbs. It felt important to remember.

Then too, I feel sensitive to touch. Now that things have opened up and I venture out more, there are fleeting touches, though rarely. This morning, I bought bread at the bakery and the woman working behind the counter brushed my hand as she gave me change. I felt her touch buzzing in my palm afterwards.

One morning, maybe in May, I went for a run and afterwards I lay down in a small field—more of an overgrown patch of grass. It smelled delicious of earth and green. The ground against my back felt good, literally grounding. Suddenly, the wind picked up and I could feel the breeze move across my skin touching me. I wept with some mix of pleasure and loneliness that I cannot really describe.

In the forensic lab, we handled bones carefully because they are fragile and easily damaged. But we are fragile too. Infection travels through touch and human remains are potential vectors of pathogens.

A friend in Buenos Aires says that people are meeting at clandestine milongas, to dance tango secretly. Other friends in Berlin have started giving tango classes again. In Paris, I see photos of people dancing in front of the Opera Garnier. I feel angry. I think these dancers are being reckless and selfish. What could be worse than tango, literally dancing cheek to cheek? But this anger is impure, because it is shot through with jealousy. I want to be among them.

In the cruel experiments that we've all read about in textbooks, when baby monkeys are presented with a metal wire frame and bottle they prefer to go hungry in the arms of a plush mother. Skin hunger will drive me to take risks eventually (Figs. 1.11 and 1.12).

Alexa Hagerty

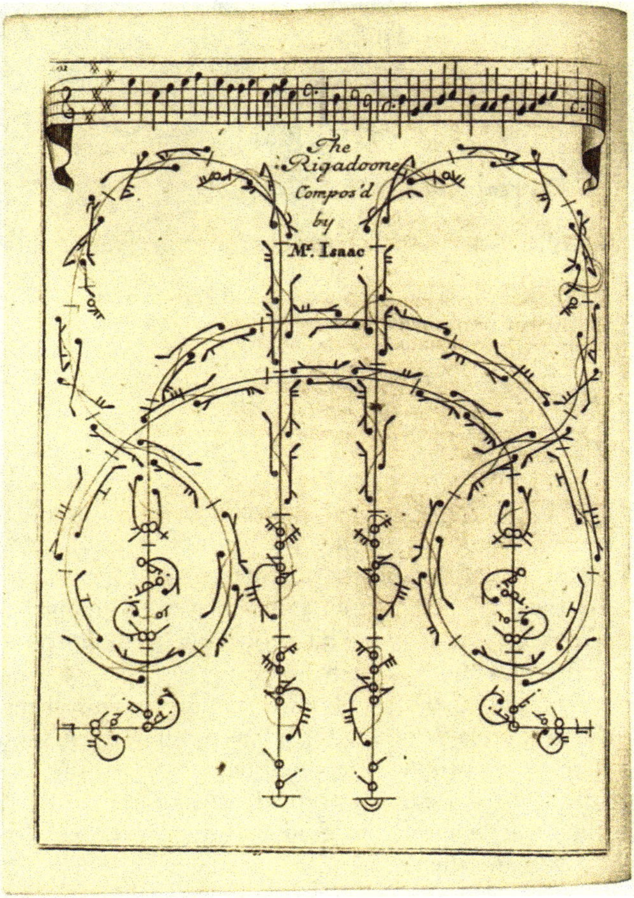

Fig. 1.11 Feuillet dance notation for a rigadoon by Isaac, first published in *Orchesography or the Art of Dancing … an Exact and Just Translation from the French of Monsieur Feuillet. By John Weaver, Dancing Master.* Second edition. London, ca. 1721. (Photo Credit: Public Domain Review)

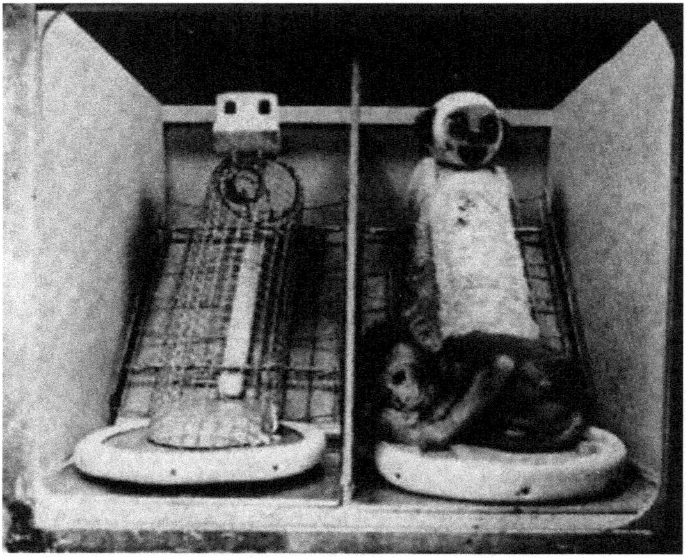

Fig. 1.12 Wire and cloth mother surrogates, 1958. (Photo by Harry Harlow, CC0, via Wikimedia Commons)

Gentle Exile

Copenhagen, August 2020.

Everything is a little bit off.

It's strange to see baseball being played again. It doesn't seem real, more like simulations of the actual game, with players going through the motions for the sake of the show. The other night Robert watched a few highlights on the ESPN.com, from games played the night before. In a win for the Yankees, Aaron Judge hit a towering homer into the left field seats. The first replay showed the ball zipping past the fence and landing into a crowd of fans in the stands as ribald Bronx fans cheered, leapt, rejoiced. The next replay, of the same home run trajectory, showed those same stands empty of people. The visual technology of the first film clip had apparently inserted a simulated crowd into a nearly vacant stadium. In this pandemic summer, sports field an odd mix of the familiar and the strange, the actual and the virtual.

Adjustments, contingency plans. Intensities and diminishments. States of stuckness, displacement. Viral contagions. A flow of intensities, movements, lines of flight, and severed lines of flight. Different temporalities and historicities clime the world. Just now, one place in North America is back in March, while another has jumped into the fall, and then life in August suddenly swivels back into how life and death were in early April. Copenhagen could easily slide back into mid-March if people aren't careful.

Everything is "in parentheses," says Q. He has been trying to plan for courses that he will supposedly teach in the fall at the University of Copenhagen. "One has to make three separate plans for each course," he said, "and that takes a lot of work. It's maddening."

In his own quadrant of experience Robert finds that he is stuck in Denmark, caught in a bureaucratic limbo that involves two or three sovereign states. He decided to stay on in Denmark this summer, once it became clear that the travel ban imposed on persons coming the United States was going into effect in early July; if he had returned to New York, as planned, he might not have been able to get back to Europe when he needed to. He is currently waiting on a visa, to be issued by the Embassy of France, in Copenhagen, which he hopes to use to get him legally to France, where a fellowship at a research institute in Paris awaits, starting in September. But for that visa to come through Robert first needs to receive an extension of his residence permit for Denmark, and report this legal fact to the French consulate. Without that confirming, necessary document, he cannot travel to France, or stay legally in Denmark. Robert's first residence permit expired in July, and while he applied for an extension to the permit at that time, he has received no word or determination from the relevant offices in Denmark. The news on that could come any day, or weeks from now.

Robert can't reach the persons and agencies involved. He cannot reach the office of immigration and speak directly with the law. He writes messages on the website server, within the rhetoric of desperate messages, but receives only automated responses.

Robert is waiting, waiting, in exilic privilege. White detention.

A dossier is being developed on Robert's exilic experience. The dossier marks dates, moments, the infinite waiting involved, despondency.

R. likens himself to the K. of Kafka's parables, who waits for years at the gate Before the Law. Or the K. who comes to be mired for days on end in the rambling village set on the fog-riddled grounds below The Castle, inaccessible, waiting to receive an invitation to enter its grounds.

The lucky ones now are those who can travel, safely and soundly, and can move from country to country, from one nervous continent to another, with little concern about visas or having the right kind of passport, without fears of not being let into a country or having to face a two-week quarantine state, holed up in a hotel somewhere, with no access to the pool, even. Others are stuck in place, even if they are trying to reach a new job somewhere, or a study program at a university, or a loved one from whom they have been separated.

For much of his life Robert found that he could count on the relative "free pass" of a US passport, and that he could travel easily to most places in the world, at least to countries where its citizens did not hate Americans. Just hop on a plane and get the tourist visa upon arrival, passing through the manned stations of border control in a sleepless early morning. Now that sense of American exceptionalism has collapsed into fiery embers, and his chances for mobility are severely limited. He can't fault anyone for wanting to keep residents of the United States from their territories right now, especially given how badly the government and its peoples have failed in containing the virus. He simply wishes things were otherwise.

He's a mild migrant, exiled in a gentle city. It's all rather safe in Denmark, though the viral numbers have started to tick upward, the country's daily count of infections. Lots of people moving about now, vacations in France and Italy, potential super-spreaders. Aarhus is close to lock-down mode again, after a sudden rash of infections, and the government is demanding that masks be worn on the public transportation there.

Copenhagen sprang back to life in May, once the limits of the lock-down were lifted. Within days Robert watched as the once-dormant shops, restaurants, and beer halls of Vesterbro opened up, like flowers and mushrooms cropping up after a spring rainstorm. It was strange to walk in the nearby shopping mall with people in it again.

Denmark has remained calm and peaceful, to date. There is not the anger and resentment and sullen despair and mask-politics evident in other places, where the virus still circulates at a frightening pace.

The sun reached its summer apex in late June. The country's solstice celebrations were muted this year, with no collective gatherings, no burning of witches. The light of the land has been in glorious decline since then.

Robert sometimes thinks of packing it up and returning home, in despondent failure. But he knows there is not much there for him, either, in New York, or elsewhere. Through the fissures of the summer light he realizes there is a kind of existential homelessness to his plight, as pretentious as that sounds. The pandemic cuts a life down to its bare formations.

Robert's apartment in New York lies quiet and uninhabited. His car, a 2012 Volkswagen Golf, remains in a parking structure on the college campus—slowly losing its battery juice, he supposes. He has run out of the medication he takes, for mild high-blood pressure, and the CVS website notes that it does not do business in Europe. He has yet to do federal or state taxes for the year 2019. His laptop is now overused, and the key for the letter "D" is starting to come undone, it's clinging to the metal frame like a loose tooth. (Why the letter D? Detention. Delay. Despair…The key holds onto the typology of a life.) Robert is tired of working hunched over the small screen of the Thinkpad.

He does not have a reliable mailing address, just now. And then there's that lost university ID card. The minor pathos of it all is rather humorous. It's also frustrating and stressful. Especially the not knowing part, the uncertainties involved.

Robert sees couples together, and groups of friends seated along the grassy interval of Somner Boulevard, drinking cans of Carlsberg pilsner and snacking on lox salmon and rugbrød. He envies the companionship and intimacy they can count on.

Robert fights off a certain sadness, at times. He tells this to M.E. while they were talking the other day by Skype, Seattle to Copenhagen. M.E. says she feels much the same, most days. When the sadness hovers she finds herself shaking her head, to shake the funk out of her thoughts. This gesture works, for a while.

In one of her recent podcasts, Michelle Obama said that she was experiencing "low-grade depression." She seemed to suggest that it was "because of a combination of quarantine, racial unrest and the Trump administration's response to the pandemic," as the New York Times put it.[30] Robert can relate to this, as can others, no doubt.

Emotionally exhausted. Stunned.

Robert learns that his first name, when pronounced in Danish, sounds something like "(R)ob(e)art." He hears this name being sounded in restaurants where he has placed an order for food; the first few times that name was called out he did not realize that he was the one being summoned. He has come to find the newly pronounced form of the name fitting for these times. The sounds are a little off, in guttural vocality, cued differently.

For lack of much else to do Robert works a lot. Writing, writing, reading, rewriting. He tells himself and others that he is working on a book manuscript. He has been working through these splendid summer days; on the weekends, too. He finds it difficult to relax or have much fun while on his own. He has not been exploring the city like he used to, back in the spring. But, all work and no play.

Robert prefers not to work in the one-room apartment that now passes as home. When he tries to do that the silence and isolation all too easily creep in. He works in cafes, mostly, or at a community center down the street—a one-time Lutheran church revamped for meaningful social life and communal *hygge*—a place that he has come to appreciate, like others who live in the neighborhood. If he gets there early enough in the morning chances are that he can snag one of the few desk-like tables set along the balcony on the second floor and write while facing a stained-glass window. Alone, among others, suffices, for now.

If Robert is away from people for too long, he forgets that they have volume. And then, when he is back in the mix of the city, he notices the depths of people, and the surfaces, so different from the visual flatness of characters on Netflix. *Best new movies to watch in July.*

Most days he treats himself to a cappuccino, and this while at Prolog, a café in the former meatpacking district, a caffeine mecca for latte-loving Vesterbro residents and beyond, at hipster-rich prices. He admires the way that the baristas prepare their drinks with skilled care and espresso virtuosity. It's surprising that the taste of a cappuccino can be so sublime, that delicate mix of espresso and milk, and he savors those few sweet moments in an afternoon when he can sip on the elixir while reading, or writing, or listening to *Keith Jarrett at the Blue Note*, on Spotify.

"Every gesture is beautiful," he thinks and realizes while seated at a side table at Prolog, watching the flow of life pass by, parents pushing their children in bike carts, the light grace of a café worker, or that bearded man who comes each morning with his dog. (Robert takes the latter for a musician, or a nightclub owner, but all that must be a mirage.)

One afternoon Robert exchanges hellos with one of the baristas working at the café. Are you going on a vacation this summer?" N asks him. No, he's not. And yourself? "No, I don't think so. We're short-staffed right now and I thought I would pick up some extra hours." They agree that the summer in Europe is different this year, in many ways. "It's strange." "It's strange."

They are all just waiting for the damn thing to be over.

An effective vaccination and resultant collective immunity are the great promise now. It's just a matter of time, or so they hope. Billions invested in that cause. They're banking on next spring or so, around March or April 2021, is one guess. But governments could mess that up, too.

Robert has yet to wear a mask in public. He wonders what that would be like. H. has told him __

Every gesture is beautiful, perhaps. Hold onto that.

(R)ob(e)art is here.
ʁo:bɐd
Robert wonders if something is a little bit off with him.

Robert Desjarlais

Dancing *With* in COVID-19

They came south by bus from Harlem and the Bronx, east by bike and subway from Brooklyn, and south-east by car from Queens. Forty or so walked through a mosquito ridden field to reach this beach bunker where grass meets sea. The first dance party any of them had attended since early Marc: a crisis dance in a world of meltdown. Any other year, you would have found them sharing cigarettes, drinking out of the same cups, conversing with strangers, dancing close. Yet COVID concerns and a storm that had moved through the city the day before, leaving some neighborhoods without electricity, deterred some from making the trek that afternoon.

I had come early to sweep out the bunker and to help Adam and his co-conspirators set up. The sun had come out. We lay sprawled on towels in small groups, a few feet apart, scattered across the small stretch of beach that felt like ours. Some dancing at the water's edge, others chatting some feet apart in the oily waters of this New York Bay, soulful electronic music flying out of the windowless windows. The bunker's expansive interior remained nearly empty for much of the afternoon, one or two masked dancers swaying within the confines of chalk circles etched onto the concrete floor. A glittery disco ball hung loose from the steel ramparts refracting the mud and grass creeping in from the four corners of the room. Two teenagers from south Brooklyn on a hike had wandered into the bunker, a young family of four splashed in the shoals, three middle-aged men fished from the concrete blocks at the water's edge.

And when the disco ball was taken down at 9:00 p.m. the dancers slowly began to disperse from whence they'd come. Three of us rode down the tarmac, arms outstretched—reaching wide—the fresh air on our faces, potholes, and fireflies accompanying us away from the bunker and back onto Flatbush Ave.

Only one week before, the New York Post published a scorching exposé blasting dancers and partygoers who had found one another under the Kosciuszko Bridge in north Brooklyn after a Black Lives Matter protest.

Hundreds Gather for Secret Rave under NYC's Kosciuszko Bridge

An illicit rave took place under the Kosciuszko Bridge in Brooklyn Saturday night, as bars and clubs remain on lockdown from the coronavirus.

Some revelers wore masks at the wild dance party that rocked into the early hours of Sunday, but showed a rampant disregard for social distancing guidelines, according to footage circulating on social media.

A crowd of hundreds could be seen at the unauthorized rave in Greenpoint, grooving to beats spun by DJ Mazurbate—who was behind a turntable setup wearing a surgical mask and bopping his head.[31]

Critical and alarming—perfect click-bait material. By far the most popular dance floor that spring and summer was on St. James Place in Clinton Hill, a block party begun by one family as a celebration of essential workers every night at 7:00 p.m.. Adam had been to the block party before and invited me to come, and so I cycled over, along with Fern, my roommate, the person I had spent every day of the last six months. Four speakers, one hour of dancing in a mask. In the *Gothamist*, Gail Bryan-Vill, who initiated the nightly dance, noted: "We're all spiritual beings, just having a human experience," adding, that we all need "a Covid-release."[32] Strangers united by dance and a remixed version of Earth Wind, and Fire's "Never" (Jay "Sinister" Full Effect). Bbounce, twirl, swish from side to side. Close your eyes. Pump your arms up and out, twist your hips, tap your feet, shake your head, feel the collective sigh of release, the ecstasy of a body in sync with strangers on a random block of Brooklyn brownstones—a release that dinner with Fern on the stoop, a walk through Prospect Park, or dancing *alone* in your Brooklyn bedroom between the dresser and the desk simply cannot offer.

The desire to dance *with* is—of course—not limited to Brooklyn. In June, the online cinema platform V-Drome introduced Jorge Jácome's "Fiesta Forever" (2016) in the following way:

> Nightlife is over, discos are ruins, a world is gone. Melancholy seems the only option. A tribute to four legendary abandoned nightclubs in Portugal presents a moving vision of the power of togetherness. Beyond walls, dance is a revolution that cannot be stopped. We just need to remember *how we feel* [emphasis mine].[33]

Watching "Fiesta Forever" during a global pandemic, four years after its release, resonates differently. This short film is a haptic encounter attuned to the frequencies and reverberations of "being on a dance floor full of people." In refusing to include visuals of dancers, the film foregrounds *sensing* the pulse, the rhythm, the repetition of the dancing body.

In his V-Drome interview with Jácome, the Spanish film curator Garbiñe Ortega describes the power of "a group of bodies in movement, bodies dancing just like one." He cites a text written by Spanish dancer Aimar Pérez Galí, "La comunidad sudorosa" (The Sweaty Community).[34]

> To soak a T-shirt with sweat isn't something one does isolated, even if they are the only one dancing. The sweat that impregnates that T-shirt is loaded with many other things, it is the result of a story that links a web of active agents that produces the feeling so that the body, motivated and involved, perspires.

To spin, dip, groove, to soak your T-shirt with sweat is to tap into the "sweaty community," to activate it each and every time. For Pérez Galí, the dancing body evokes Victor Turner's *communitas,* "an unstructured rudimentary community that emerges in the liminal period of social drama."[35] To dance is to be many bodies in one, enabling dancers to bend the rules of social relations and to invoke a "community in singularity."[36]

While in Paris in early October, I was listening to one of philosopher Géraldine Mosna-Savoye's brief programs for French radio. In reflecting on the pandemic and her desire to be with others, she made droll remarks about her nostalgia for parties. A wave of emotion overcame her as she sipped her tea, the nightly "COVID news" in the background, a "lonely spectator" observing a group of masked colleagues in the building across the way—reckless, enjoying themselves, singing Céline Dion's *Pour que tu m'aimes encore* at the top of their lungs. Was it not, she asks, Emile Durkheim in the *Elementary Forms of Religious Life* who spoke of that which cannot be reduced to being several, a collection of individual selves? Of how "ways of acting or thinking" taken collectively "take on a body, a sensible form that is specific to them, and constitutes a reality *sui generis*, distinct from the individual facts that manifest it."[37] Of course, she says, we can create solidarity on an individual level, but to dine with a couple of friends has literally nothing to do with a party of twenty. What, she asks, "remains of these collective ways that go beyond us, where we forget ourselves, where we do not theorize a 'we,' a 'living together,' but where we are quite simply together?"

Durkheim and Turner's concepts emerged out of an analysis of initiation rites—events closely associated with dance ceremonies and saturated with myth, the occult, and the vitality of the crowd. The beach bunker, the Kosciuszko bridge, and the block party were sites of a collective corporeal release. They were an invitation, a small offering in the present, to a future in which the fear of entangled bodies would be no more. In this modern western world where rituals are few and far between, do these COVID dances take on an extra intensity? An anti-structural moment, as Turner would call it, which receives its meaning—and its feeling—from the structure that it holds at bay *or* is it simply the body, the music, and the big empty sky?

Margaux Fitoussi

Notes

1. Yurchak (2005).
2. Davis (2020).
3. Freud (1955:151–318).

4. For a full text of Trump's oval address of March 11, 2020, see https://www.nytimes.com/2020/03/11/us/politics/trump-coronavirus-speech.html (last accessed, April 3, 2022).
5. https://travel.state.gov/content/travel/en/international-travel/International-Travel-Country-Information-Pages/Italy.html (last accessed July 3, 2020).
6. I am referring here to the diplomatic tensions following the US assassination of Iranian General Qasem Soleimani, in early January 2020. https://www.nytimes.com/2020/01/05/us/politics/iranian-americans-border.html (last accessed, April 3, 2022).
7. https://www.npr.org/sections/goatsandsoda/2020/03/12/814876173/coronavirus-trump-speech-creates-chaos-eu-says-it-wasnt-warned-of-travel-ban (last accessed, April 3, 2022).
8. https://twitter.com/profviolence/status/1239138646076329984 (last accessed, April 3, 2022).
9. As Benjamin (1999 [N9, 7]: 473) highlights in his unfinished *Arcades Project*, historical intelligibility is afforded by dialectical images, which "emerge suddenly in a flash," interrupting the continuity of temporal succession by bringing together the now and the once has been and making historical time legible.
10. See: https://www.youtube.com/watch?v=8sx0zRbHAbM; or https://www.youtube.com/watch?v=46wvy-64fS0
11. See here: https://www.nytimes.com/2020/04/30/nyregion/coronavirus-nyc-funeral-home-morgue-bodies.html
12. Desjarlais (2011, 2021).
13. The radical nationwide-lockdown established by executive decrees of March 11 and March 22, 2020 was followed by a partial reopening on May 4 and further expanded by the Decree Law number 33 of May 16, 2020, which went into effect on May 18.
14. "Corona virus can live on asphalt for up to nine days," stated an alarmist WhatsApp message form an unverified source, generating panic among the Italian population throughout the month of March. The news was later disproved as fake, see Alessia Strinati's article on *Il Mattino*, March 16, 2020.

    https://www.ilmattino.it/societa/persone/coronavirus_sopravvive_asfalto_scarpe_fake_news_ultime_notizie_oggi_16_marzo_2020-5114056.html (last accessed, April 3, 2022).
15. WhatsApp message with Luca Ciabarri, May 22, 2020.
16. Decree Law number 33 of May 16, 2020.
17. The Decree Law of March 11 extended to the entire country the lockdown that had been originally only applied to small towns in Veneto and Lombardy (Decree Law of February 22). During the night between March

7 and 8, a more extensive decree was prepared with the aim of implementing further restrictions and curb domestic travel across regions. A draft of the decree, however, was leaked and circulated widely on social networks, causing a wave of panic among the many southern Italians working in the more industrialized regions of the country's North. The fear of remaining stranded away from their families prompted them to rush to the nearest station and catch "the last train south." As a response to the exodus and to its potential negative effects on the spreading of the virus in the southern regions, the government issued the #Istayathome decree, initiating the first COVID-related nation-wide lockdown in the world.

18. Public parks remained inaccessible until the beginning of phase 2, which started on May 4.
19. *La Repubblica*, April 17, 2020. https://milano.repubblica.it/cronaca/2020/04/17/news/coronavirus_lombardia_in_giro_ben_pettinato_a_rovellasca_multa_per_lui_e_il_parucchiere-254275740/ (last accessed, April 3, 2022).
20. April 14, 2020, *Il mattino.it.* https://www.ilmattino.it/primopiano/cronaca/moglie_bagagliaio_sfuggire_controlli_casa_mare-5170584.html (last accessed, April 3, 2022).
21. April 15, 2020, Blogsicilia.it https://www.blogsicilia.it/palermo/passeggia-in-viale-regione-siciliana-con-la-pecora-al-guinzaglio-multato-a-palermo-video/529599/(last accessed, April 3, 2022).
22. Povinelli (2006: 10).
23. See Decree Law of April 26, 2020.
24. For a legal dissertation, in Italian, on the notion of "congiunti" see Francesco Meglio, April 28, 2020, *La nozione di «congiunti» e il D.P.C.M. 26 aprile 2020.*
    http://www.rivistafamilia.it/2020/04/28/la-nozione-congiunti-d-p-c-m-26-aprile-2020/(last accessed, April 3, 2022).
25. WhatsApp message with Chiara Martucci, May 4, 2020.
26. Prior to Independence in 1963 and the formation of Malaysia, the Federation of Malaya encompassed the 11 peninsular states, including Singapore, Penang, and Malacca.
27. My analysis here echoes Martha Kaplan's approach to the semiotics of Fiji water circulating in the New York (Kaplan 2007).
28. Way (2020).
29. Wong et al. (2011).
30. Taylor, Derrick Bryson. "Michelle Obama Says She is Dealing with 'Low-Grade Depression'." New York Times August 6, 2020 (https://www.nytimes.com/2020/08/06/us/michelle-obama-depression.html; last accessed May 16, 2022).

31. Rosner, Elizabeth. "Hundreds Gather for Secret Rave under NYC's Kosciuszko Bridge." New York Post (https://nypost.com/2020/08/03/hundreds-gather-for-secret-rave-under-nycs-kosciuszko-bridge/; last accessed May 16, 2022).
32. Carlson, Jen. "Video: How Brooklyn's Biggest 7 O'Clock 'Covid-Release Block Party' Began." Gothamist (https://gothamist.com/arts-entertainment/video-how-brooklyns-biggest-7-oclock-covid-release-block-party-began; last accessed May 16, 2022).
33. Ibid.
34. Ibid. Galí published a book "Sudando el discourso" (Sweating the Discourse, 2013) that accompanied this work in July 2015 with the support of Mar Medina, Paul B. Preciado, Jaime Conde-Salazar and the sweaty community.
35. Jacomé, Jorge, and Garbiñe Ortega. "Jorge Jácome 'Fiesta Forever.'" *Interview,* V-Drome.
36. Ibid.
37. Mosna-Savoye (2020), who cites Durkheim (1912).

CHAPTER 2

Part II: The Second Wave

We are all now invited to write the next series of entries using the method of a modified "exquisite corpse." For the French surrealists, among other artists, the cadaver exquis—literally, "exquisite cadaver"—entailed a technique by which a collection of words or images is collectively assembled. Each collaborator adds to a composition in sequence, according to a certain rule or method, or by being allowed to see only the end of what a previous person has contributed—such as a sequence of writing, or a drawing being composed, step by step. For our purposes here, we have agreed to proceed with a sequence of contributions, with each entry crafted by someone following the words of another. Each new contributor has three days to complete and send along their text—the next contribution to the collective writing, that is—and then the writing moves on to the next contributor, and so on, until everyone has had a chance to contribute. (Anyone can take a "pass" when it's their turn, if they so wish to...)
September 2020

"It's Covidtastic"

The despair is back. It's in the apartment now, lurking. There is that pitch-dark hole in the drain of the bathroom sink, and the raven gloom of dress shoes to the far side of the closet. A charcoal-coated suitcase lies closed and empty. Gray, cement-like floors. Obscure depths of a microwave oven.

R. Desjarlais et al., *Dispatches from Home and the Field during the COVID-19 Pandemic*, Palgrave Studies in Literary Anthropology,
https://doi.org/10.1007/978-3-031-19193-0_2

The oily glass sheen of my cell phone when unlit is unnerving. I try not to look at it directly, though that void catches my eye. I have to be careful. I try not to think about it too much. It's there waiting for me when I wake up. Oblivion while asleep, and then it all resurfaces again. The days are getting shorter now. When I wake up there is only the briefest of light. I find myself searching for the clearest of blue skies.

This past Sunday we were informed that we would not be able to work this week at the institute in Paris where I am now a research fellow. Someone who works there was notified that she or he had been in contact with someone who had tested positive for the virus. Two degrees of separation—or possible contagion. We are now waiting for the results of the test that the second person received. With this I am now into day three of dreary lunches and nonsocial hours. Swirling recesses of toil and delay in the drab solitude of a makeshift "home" brings fugue memories of last spring, when there were months of confinement, aloneness, zoom soliloquies, uncertain fears, night-long viewings of Nordic noir.

Each novel fold of a week brings unexpected permutations of safety, risk, sanitary protocols, global charts, and infection rates. Vectors of time and space constantly take new forms. Each week offers an unstable horizon on any new possibilities, impossibilities, ruptures, breakdown promises. Each inscription in time would need to be updated in a fortnight, to account for a multitude of shifts in contagion rates, death counts, governmental mandates, restrictions, or the prospect of new medicines or vaccines. On this, our thinking is vague.

"I don't know what is true and not true anymore," said a friend a few days back. She was speaking about the oscillating statements of public health experts and governmental officials in France the past few months. "They've said so many things, since March, and they keep changing their minds."

We sat on the grass of a sloping hill near one of the ponds in Parc de Buttes Chaumont, the Sunday of the national *Journées du Patrimoine* (Days of Heritage). Three young men were tossing a football around. Like others enjoying the park that day, we sought out pockets of normalcy, warm and fleeting exchanges, sunlight, while aware of the risks of being in public and semi-conscious of any possible, encroaching second wave.

We watched Isabelle's daughter Nadège play with some newly made friends around her age, the games led by their mother or caretaker. In the throes of a game of tag, French-style, the woman lightly tapped the top of Nadège's head. "Oh," Isabelle said. "She's not supposed to do that. She's not supposed to touch other people—outside her family." She looked upon the scene of play, monitoring the gestures, as if she was giving thought to saying something. She looked away, and said, "Oh well...."

At a nervous gathering the other day, an impromptu apéro among other research fellows of the institute here, at our place of collective residence, a building set on a residential campus at the southern edge of the city, we stood on a terrace outside, five flights up, facing a cold brisk wind, and the threat of pelting rain. We held glasses of wine in our hands. We were glad to be among these new acquaintances of ours, talking, smiling, while not wanting to get too close. We didn't know whether to keep our masks on, or not. One man, the eldest, arrived wearing a plastic face guard, which he soon put to the side.

It got colder still, and we moved inside, huddled in the kitchen. The conversation turned to the pandemic. Our host, an art historian, looked around, catching the thoughts of each person there, and said, "Chances are that one of us here will get it. It's almost certain to happen."

"Yeah," I chipped in. "It will be like one of those murder mysteries, set in a spooky house or a deserted island—'And then there was one!'"

No one laughed.

We were standing on a precipice.

We turned to those next to us and chatted anew. We sipped from glasses of Bourgogne and snacked on sliced carrots, chips, and hummus. A six-year-old girl came to the counter, smiled, and tasted some of the hors d'œuvres.

"Yum!" she said with a laugh. "It's Covidtastic!"

"It's Covidtastic?! Did you come up with this word?" I asked.

The girl smiled.

All of these permutations in thought and life and joy and anxious fear and fantastic concern, and a child's linguistic play, took place before the despair began to seep, again.

We are waiting for the test results to come in.

Could be any day, now.

Robert Desjarlais

The Morning Commute

Despair is never far away. Second, third, and fourth waves, surges and resurgences, additional super-spreader events, intensifying neighborhood clusters, proliferating "red zones," maps of new cases trending upwards, again.

Despite my ritualized digestion of the latest updates and an overcast sky on this Friday morning, the gloom that has marked much of this year for so many does not seem to capture the mood on the sidewalk. Instead, it feels busy. As I take my children to school, a mother and two daughters rush by, clearly late for class. A few steps later, I wheel the stroller around a slow walker and two texters. Crossing-guards who weeks earlier were often on their phones this morning are in the intersections helping others make their way across the streets. In the summer, especially in late afternoons on hot days, the sidewalks had been filled with people looking to wander, exercise, and connect. But this morning, as public schools enter their third week of (partial) operation, and daycares and private and parochial schools continue their staggered re-openings, I am struck by the feeling we are in a new phase with a different energy: The return of the morning school-work commute. It feels tentative, hopeful, and familiar.

Four weeks later, I return to this post. The editors of our collaborative project have asked each of us to revise our entries—in my case, to expand my reflection so that it can better co-exist with the longer entries that followed. I have been putting it off. Part of my hesitation comes from wanting to avoid revisiting what I wrote. The October morning commute feels far away, an isolated experience perhaps not worth preserving.

Moreover, its optimism today seems misplaced. With the exception of the brief pleasure of spontaneous, public celebrations of the Biden-Harris victory on a glorious, sunny Saturday, I recently have been reckoning with the grim realization that a new wave is coming back to New York. When did this future come to feel inevitable? Maybe it was last week when the country first broke the threshold of 100,000 daily infections. Or perhaps it was during a conversation I had with a restaurant owner who explained that after watching developments in Europe she had already decided to forgo putting more money into her COVID-era outdoor eating spaces. It could have been at a meeting this week where colleagues expressed doubts about our university's re-opening plans. Or maybe it came with the grim jokes my wife and I have been making about the inevitably of our son's daycare closing given other families' resistance to mask policies.

I find my thoughts spinning as I turn to the looming prospect of more virtual classes, more quarantining, and more of that awful feeling of the Spring when the virus seemed to be everywhere. While I am writing this, my phone lights up. The mayor has announced schools could close as early as Monday—the positivity rate keeps going up. It just won't stop.

Nicholas Bartlett

Toothpaste

I had underestimated the side effects of the quarantine. After months of hardcore lockdown in Milan, what would a couple of weeks of self-isolation in my NYC apartment do? I arrived on a Thursday, after crossing the Atlantic on a nearly empty Delta flight—a forced return not to lose my status as a lawful permanent resident. The robocall I received two days after my arrival confirmed the already known: I had to separate from other people and stay at my residence all the time. A flurry of identical text messages ensued, reinforcing the unequivocal injunction by the automated voice call and requesting I confirm I had understood the judicial implications and potential ramifications for violating the travel advisory that Governor Cuomo issued at the beginning of the summer:

> THIS IS A MESSAGE FROM THE NEW YORK CITY TEST & TRACE CORPS para ver esta mesaje en espanol presione E. You recently traveled to NYC from a state with a high rate of COVID-19. State law REQUIRES that you quarantine for 14 days from the day you left that state. You are required to stay inside your home and only leave for critical needs like medical care. Please call 844-692-4692, if you cannot safely quarantine from others in your home, or if you develop symptoms of COVID and cannot speak to your medical provider. The City can help you! If this is an emergency, call 911. Please confirm you understand your obligations under state law by responding to this text with the letter 'C'. Msg & Data Rates May Apply

The autocratic robotic voice and the vibration pulses of the text message ripple the amorphous silence in my apartment, interrupting my apathetic numbness and throwing me in a state of inexplicable panic. I scramble to respond to the prompt by swiftly typing the letter "C" in the message body. I receive another text:

Thank you for your response.

My compliance does not grant me the expected relief. I am startled by another burst of sinister vibrations. I grab my phone, a quasi-identical message:

THIS IS AN IMPORTANT MESSAGE FROM THE NEW YORK CITY TEST & TRACE CORPS.... You recently traveled to NYC from a state with a high rate of COVID-19. State law REQUIRES that you quarantine for 14 days .... only leave for critical needs like medical care....The

City can help you! ... Please confirm you understand your obligations under state law by responding to this text with the letter 'C'....

— C

Thank you for your response.

I receive another text:

THIS IS A MESSAGE FROM THE NEW YORK CITY TEST & TRACE CORPS para ver esta mesaje en espanol presione E. ... State law REQUIRES that you ... stay inside your home... Please call 844-692-4692, if you cannot safely quarantine from others in your home, or if you develop symptoms of COVID and cannot speak to your medical provider... Please confirm you understand your obligations ... Msg & Data Rates May Apply

— C

Thank you for your response.

Another text, and then another. I start wondering what would happen if I were to press "E" for Spanish. Would the notifications stop? What letter would I be required to type to confirm I understand my obligations under state law in the Spanish version of this message? I am tempted to try. But I refrain myself. It would be too subversive a gesture to play with the notifications from the New York City Test & Trace Corps.

As my quarantine days go by, the texts continue, but my reactions subside. I notice that each new message startles me less and less. Am I getting used to the new routine? The texts no longer surprise me. Unable to focus, I listen to the news about the spreading of new cluster outbreaks in Europe. I feel dizzy, muddled. But I no longer experience the gripping bursts of fear that punctuated my days during the first wave. I wonder if I have lost my capacity for awe.

I linger in my apartment in a state of lethargic anxiety. This state of emergency has become a deafening white noise—a flat acoustic presence that saturates our sonic imagination with a fuzzy blend of all audible frequencies. Its constant spectral density fills my apartment, making it impossible to imagine an elsewhere. Oh, how I wish I could float out of this endless suspension! Perhaps, I could productively use the time to "declutter"? I soon find myself drifting through the contents of my apartment. Forgotten objects reappear, bringing back memories of a time past, opening up wormhole passages to a different me. I try to listen to the stories that I know are recorded in the objects now scattered on the floor, but their voices are muffled by the same white noise that saturates my apartment. I am overwhelmed by a creeping sense of estrangement from my own belongings. The affective memories they evoke feel like someone else's. I am haunted by the thought of the implanted memories of androids.

Perhaps I am becoming (or have always been) one? My mind goes to a classic dystopian cyberpunk scene. “You think I am a replicant don’t you?” asks Rachel as she seeks to convince blade runner agent Deckard that she is human by sharing with him detailed private memories of her childhood. Deckard interrupts her narrative to recall to her the memories of her own childhood: “Implants! Those aren’t your memories, they are somebody else’s. That’s all, just implants.” As Rachel starts to cry, quietly, Deckard is moved to compassion and clumsily tries to remediate: “O.K., bad joke... I made a bad joke. You’re not a replicant.”

As I sit alone alienated from my own objects and no longer capable of shedding tears I wonder whether I, too, am only a sophisticated android convinced of being human. In search of an escape from the dissociative metamorphic effects of the quarantine, I cling to my aluminum toothpaste tube (Fig. 2.1). Every time I squeeze out a quantum of product, its aluminum body takes a slightly different new shape—providing me with a material trace of the passing of these endless days, like an irreversible hourglass of sorts.

Aurora Donzelli

Fig. 2.1 Aluminum toothpaste tube turned hourglass. (Photo by A. Donzelli)

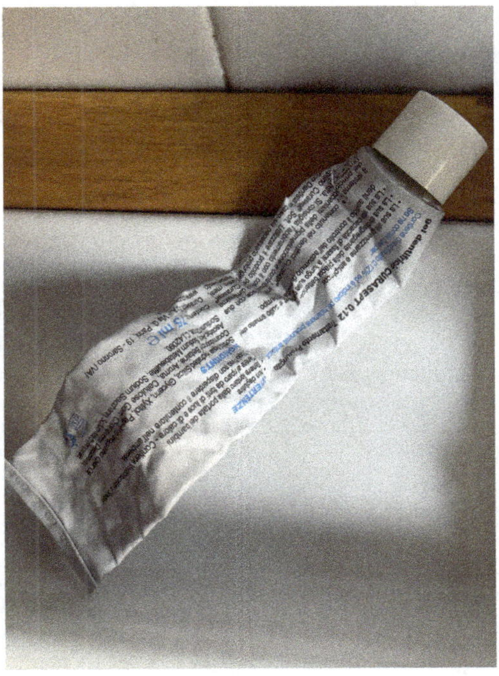

DiCTATURe eN COURS

The night the curfew went into place, a *jeu de mots* appeared on the walls of my neighborhood in northeast Paris. *DiCTATURe eN COURS* scrawled in black ink on the walls of the Franprix, the Belleville Cemetery, and the tanning salon across the street from my flat. The same hasty script, the same black letters. The consonants *angry*, the vowels slightly hesitant. DiCTATURe eN COURS meaning DICTATORSHIP IN PROGRESS or DICTATORSHIP IN THE CLASSROOM.

The next day I walked up Rue de Télégraph on the way to my aunt's for shabbat lunch. MACRONAVIRUS stenciled in white on the sidewalk in front of her apartment. My cousins were late, and so my aunt decided we would start without the men, passing around my favorite Tunisian kémia—mekbouba, slata mechouia, and batata haimi—while speaking to me and her daughters through her black mask. My cousin and I had cleared the table and then walked up two flights of stairs to the storage space that had become her bedroom. Laying side by side on her twin bed, the walls close around us, she told me about packing her bag and leaving her husband as soon as she heard about the lockdown. She hadn't thought twice. Afraid of what the coming months would be like, alone, in a tiny apartment with a volatile man who had hurt her before. I sat in her small room, and listened to her speak for several hours. I hadn't meant to stay so long. It had been over a year since I had seen her, and what a year it had been. I walked home at a quick clip. Nearly home, nearly curfew. At the corner of Place des Fêtes, I glanced down, LE MONDE EST AUSSI À #NOUSTOUTES stamped in pink. *Nous Toutes:* a feminist collective committed to ending sexist and sexual violence in France.

Black, white, and pink markings on the walls and sidewalks of Paris—*DiCTATURe eN COURS*, MACRONAVIRUS, LE MONDE EST AUSSI À #NOUSTOUTES—traces that interrupt our everyday, asking us to reckon with the political and intimate violence exacerbated by the pandemic (Fig. 2.2).

Margaux Fitoussi

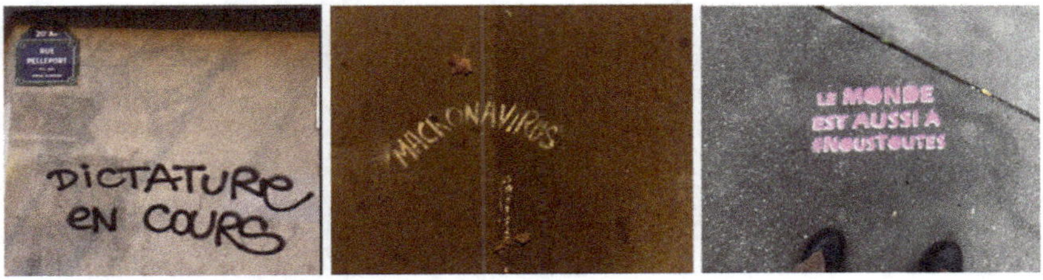

Fig. 2.2 Graffiti in the streets of Paris. (Photo by M. Fitoussi)

How Everything Can Collapse

I am taking a photograph of the theater when I notice the first protester at the periphery of my lens. After weeks of wearing a groove between the house I am renting, the park where I run, and the grocery stores where I quickly shop, I have ventured to a nearby town, in Occitanie, France.

On the train ride I listened to a podcast discussing the risk of the total collapse of industrial civilization due to climate crisis, fossil fuel dependence, and erosion of democracy. In France, collapsologie is a veritable movement, discussed by public intellectuals, debated by philosophers, sparked by a 2015 book *Comment tout peut s'effondrer* / How everything can collapse.

I get off the train, my head full of collapse, and walk into town. On Sundays in small town France almost everything closes. Maybe at some other moment the quiet buildings and empty streets would feel peaceful but today everything feels post-apocalyptic: the shuttered shops, the boarded-up windows, the bored menace of teenage boys leaning on a wall in front of the town's famous Cathedral, the tin bullets of nitrous oxide littering the sidewalk.

But the southern light is beautiful. I take photos of ramshackle buildings, framing the shot to capture the light and leave out the dark mood. This editorial trick is for no one but myself and my urge to rewrite my day in a more hopeful register.

The masked protesters turn the street corner onto the main square, loosely gathering in front of the theater steps. Two masked police officers shamble behind them. It is a protest, the signs and banners attest to that, but it doesn't feel like one. It is sedate, almost listless. Nothing like protests in Paris pulsing from Place de la République, ebullient or angry, but never flat. I walk closer to get a better view. The first sign I see says "*Je veux pouvoir enseigner sans ensaigner*" ("I want to be able to teach without bleeding"). Later, on the news I will see footage of protests all over the country, and they will be narrated as defiant crowds and a unified nation. But in this town, I feel something more like resignation and palpable exhaustion.

In collapsologie, catastrophes are often described as "interlinking." But I wonder if this is how it really works. Does each catastrophe retain its shape, its discrete form, like a string of firecrackers or iron links in a chain? Or do they bleed together? Rise to drowning in a numb tide?

Near this town, there's an army camp where the unmarked graves of Algerian babies have been found. The railway to Auschwitz ran through this town. This town was once the site of a massacre of a forgotten Christian sect. This town was once glorious in a vanished Empire. Before a thousand years of silt, this town stood by the sea.

Alexa Hagerty

Virtual Travels

In the summer of 2019, somewhat bored while doing field research in Indonesia, I browsed online travel guides extensively, fantasizing about all the places that I can go on a graduate student budget. Perhaps staying with some family friends in Holland could make international travel both affordable and fun in 2020. Perhaps redeeming all the airline miles I had collected could pay for domestic flights around Indonesia. After years of traveling and doing fieldwork in different places around the world, I felt confident that, no matter where I am, I can always be in motion: I can always enjoy the sight of people passing by while sitting in a bus, a train, a motorcycle taxi, or a ferry. I had fantasies that, if my career in anthropology did not result in full-time employment, I could look for jobs in the airline industry, where the opportunity to travel and talk to people I've never met before seemed limitless.

Thus, when international borders were shut down and domestic travel became heavily restricted in March 2020, I was profoundly disappointed in myself and the world—what can I do next? What can I even do as an anthropologist, whose scholarship and teaching seem to be motivated by the experience of traveling and making new acquaintances? What can I do as a travel enthusiast when a group of more than five people in a vehicle scares me?

The experience of travel defined my own relationship to the world before the pandemic, and it still does. Before, I would take public transit for two hours each way just to visit a museum or a beach at the other end of Chicago's vast urban expanse. However, in March 2020, when Chicago issued a stay-at-home order, these previously mundane forms of travel came to an abrupt halt. I lost of the ability to go places, to meet strangers and acquaintances alike, and I experienced this moment as a profound loss.

In the summer of 2020, however, I discovered something unexpected: the virtually limitless ability to see and read about new places on Google Maps. Each time a moment of exhaustion or boredom in front of a screen struck me, I would choose a city or a town to navigate virtually through the street view feature. As if navigating a new city on foot, I would pay attention to the details of local architecture, storefront signs, the traffic, and the landscape. I also discovered that I can read endless amounts of reviews and comment on local businesses—something that reminds of the richly textured narratives that I would overhear from ambient chatter in diners, roadside stalls, and coffee shops.

"Incredibly delicious.... [Even] government ministers and high-ranking officials can't get enough [of the dishes from this diner]," says a review of a nasi kapau ("rice with side dishes") establishment in Bukittinggi, a town in West Sumatra I have wanted to visit for a long time.

"The crispy cassava pieces [add] a really nice crunchy texture to the meal!" says another Google Maps reviewer, who posted a photo only a year ago.

I then navigated local streets on Google Maps' Street view—imagining the swerving scooters that would scare the nervous pedestrian in me. I turned my view towards an old building on the left—something that looks like a bungalow from the 1920s. I thought to myself: what would it look like inside? I hope I can visit the building in person one day!

To add the auditorial to the visual, I played some 1990s Malay music from the Spotify app on my computer. The accordions in the background reminded me of a great-aunt who played the accordion so skillfully, and, who died, unexpectedly, while playing her favorite instrument to an audience of happy school children on a camping trip. I listened to Siti Nurhaliza, a legendary Malaysian singer, as she sang a stanza from Kaparinyo, an old Malay song:

Semenjak lembah bertambah dalam
Nampaknya gunung tinggi bertuah
Semenjak sejarah Hawa dan Adam
Alam berkembang berubah-ubah

Ever since valleys grew deeper
It seems befitting that mountains grew taller
Ever since the story of Eve and Adam
The world keeps growing and changing

Taken from a 1997 recording, this stanza from Kaparinyo takes after the canonical structure of a Malay pantun, a poem with four lines. The last two lines tell me that, even when I do not physically travel, the world itself keeps moving. Much like the glacial pace of valleys eroding and volcanoes growing upward, I might stay still, but my relationship with distant places and distant acquaintances continues to evolve.

All of these experiences of virtual travel gave me hope: someday, I will once again rub shoulders with strangers and new acquaintances, and I will listen to their stories again—stories that enrich our shared lives as fellow human beings.

Rafadi Hakim

Rinse and Repeat

Sometimes it's tranquil, serene and peaceful. Other times it's lonely and isolated. Cocooned off from the rest of the world, the peace and quiet seem like an illusion that only suburban life in a small midwestern town in Central Illinois can provide. Strolls around the neighborhood and rides to local drive-through cafes and stores, in between commutes to the daycare, have become a daily routine that keeps us mind-numbingly occupied. Taking care of chores—cleaning, cooking, taking care of the baby, rinse, and repeat—while finding pockets of time to read students' work, prepare for classes, attend meetings and teach, pretty much takes up all of our time. It feels extremely mind-numbing, especially as time drags on and there doesn't seem to be any change in sight. Is this what most of us have come to rely upon to get through these days of limbo? The week of the election (a week!) added insult to injury, as every chore and errand were filled with quick, anxious checks of the phone for the latest update on ballots.

A friend shared a reflection earlier this month, that this is what the end of the world will actually look like—not wanton destruction, chaos, and annihilation, but people repeatedly doing the most mundane of chores with their minds turned off and with vacant stares. The end of the world will just be people strolling around their blocks and homes doing chores and nothing else. Rinse and repeat. Of course, this is likely the more privileged version of the end of the world. One for those of us who have the ability to move to pastures that are safer and stable. Maybe my friend intended to relate how he was experiencing the trials of the mundane everyday under COVID, but it made me think too of the dilemma of being fragmented and living transnationally "stretched" lives, where the everyday under COVID involves frequent check-ins and calls to another part of the world, where family and friends are trying to get through their days, their errands and chores, under very different conditions. Either way, the cold comfort of errands and chores—their relative predictability and their power of taking our minds away from whatever existential crisis we are facing collectively or individually—seems to be what makes the everyday possible at the moment.

It's hard to break out of this type of a cycle, especially when the work we normally do requires a particular type of sharpness and willingness to change constantly that routines may not help with. To spot changes, to see transformations, to be able to envision different ways and alternative models, all this requires a way of life that keeps us on our toes, rather than one that makes us set in our ways and repetitions. At least, that's how it used to be. It is going to be quite a challenge to break out of the habits we've been forming these days. As much as most of us want desperately to return to normal, the mere fact that we would be in this mode of life for more than a year makes it unlikely that we would even remember what the old normal felt like. The thought of being in a space with another human being without masks would cause discomfort. The thought of being outside, getting back to old routines, will be exhausting after a short while. Whether we like it or not, we've been forced to become homebodies—at least, those of us who aren't essential labor—and in many cases, our social circles have turned into very narrow bubbles. I see this happening now in an alarming way with the stranger anxiety our daughter is developing, and by extension ourselves, whenever we are in a new space with new people. For someone who used to love nothing more than traveling to a new place, constantly looking forward to the uncertainty of the unfamiliar, this newly developed fear and suspicion of strangers (what if they are Trump-supporters? What if they don't believe in science and think the pandemic is a hoax?? What if they didn't really sanitize the furniture and surfaces??) is going to take some time to get over.

Parthiban Muniandy

Music

Music seems always to be playing across my corner of the street. It is not new, but has it always been like this? Or is it that when the rest of the world grew still, the wavelets began to inch a little further, turning toward the reaches of my apartment?

Since Juneteenth, perhaps, something changed around Lake Merritt from the quiet of Oakland's early pandemic days. After waves of protest, solemn and furious, bursts of sound and bustle began filling the air around the calm waters. Street vendors cropped up where they hadn't before. Speakers boom from parked cars. An outdoors theater began appearing every weekend, peopling the lake into the night. Small dance parties under airy tent tops. Davido, Popcaan, the Fugees. Those who moved from East and West Africa and the Caribbean as adults. Those who moved from there as children. Those born here to parents who moved in their own younger years. Those born here through the enslavement of their kin. Those who live nearby. Those who arrived from various suburban reaches. This, as one man put it, was one of the few places, during the pandemic, where something was different. Special. Possible. Meanwhile, neighborhood complaints abound. As one woman interviewed on the local news put it, commenting on the emergence of crowds around the lake on weekends, "I do not feel comfortable coming out to the lake to even walk our dog."

"The propensity to dance in America is both corrosive and preservative, both uncountable and accumulable," Fred Moten writes. "If we embrace obscenity and contradiction, just in the way we move with them, it's not only because sometimes the terror of resisting earthly terror feels good, it's also because the terror of feeling good is not optional."[1]

Across the city, George Floyd gazes at the world from murals—murals on concrete surfaces, murals on storefronts boarded up since the protests. He could not breathe, and now he breathes from the walls. Days ago, in relative quiet, the third-degree murder charge against Derek Chauvin was dropped. Weeks ago, no charges were made against the officers who shot Breonna Taylor. What distinguishes living from breathing, and the deadliness from the vitality in each? What is it to be life-bound and death-bound with every breath—to respire toward death even as every breath scaffolds the passage through life? As I write this, the music is still playing. I think I'll go outside now.

Emily Ng

I Lost You

COVID-19 Pandemic has become a scary phrase. But our world has seen similar pandemics before, perhaps even worse ones. Although, of course, we are still in the beginning of the COVID-19 pandemic, aren't we? This means that the present pandemic could be among the worst ones. We still don't know. Everything has been so uncertain, so blurry, cloudy. This new reality infuses thoughts and sensations of fear, loss, solitude, and profound sadness. Death, moreover, has become even more palpable. It has been touching humans with more intensity not only with numbers that have been growing exponentially across the globe, but in our everyday microcosms as well. Have you seen how many lives COVID-19 has taken away in New York City?

It was your home. I lost you.

Your omnipresence has been suddenly dissipated by the last words you uttered before leaving us. Those words are still floating in the air. The virus won't be able to destroy them, to infect them, to replicate in them. It won't have that power, will it? You didn't have the time to show your suffering and your deep concerns about COVID-19. You stayed silent, with dignity, without complaining. You didn't show us your anxiety, your pain, your warm tears. You knew that you were leaving. You went away. You didn't want to see how Italy, where you were born and raised for many years, succumbed to the tentacles of COVID-19 early on in the pandemic. You just couldn't handle it. Knowing that your brother was there while you were here, in a complex, unprecedented spatiotemporal configuration, was depleting your human self. COVID-19 took you away from this suffering. It was too hard, too painful to watch. You were powerless. You couldn't change the course of events. You were thinking about your aunt during those days: like almost 500,000 Italians, she too died from the 1918-1920 Influenza. She was only 5.

You knew it. I lost you.

I miss our long, weekly phone calls in Italian, a language that you spoke eloquently until your last day. You were my protector, the one who was overseeing my American journey in a way that nobody else could have done. You, too, were a migrant to, and in, the United States. You knew the challenges, humiliations, subtle, and blatant injustices that migrants face on a daily basis. But COVID-19 doesn't care, does it? The virus doesn't show any preferences. It simply needs human cells to replicate fast and thus survive. New York, a city with many migrants from across the globe, including yourself, your home where you raised your three children, was hit hard. You didn't see it. It would have been unbearable to your heart. You were buried right before that. No funerals were allowed. You were finally reunited with Uncle Joseph. Strangers buried you. We were not allowed to accompany you on your last trip on this planet. I miss you.

Sabina M. Perrino

Working From Home

I sign off of Zoom and remove my bulky black headphones, having concluded two and a half hours of back-to-back meetings. One was as a representative on the faculty senate executive committee, the other as a mentor for graduate students meeting semi-regularly to discuss grant proposals, dissertation chapters, theoretical ideas, life.

"The Representative": Listen. Meeting's starting. No guests today so no introductions needed and on to business. Read the chat box, should I reply to that? We need to recommend people to be on a panel on microcredentials. I still don't know what they are. Will they call on me? Check email. I need to write that letter of recommendation for Amy. When is that due? I check the task list on the excel spreadsheet I made. Three days from now. Suggest people to serve on a selection committee to pick a common reading for the class of 2021. Last time it was *Between the World and Me*. Did I serve on that committee? I recommend someone who will say no. Should we invite someone from the libraries working on the anti-racism resource list? Do we know that anti-racism will be the theme? Silence. Find the last letter I wrote for Amy. Read it quickly. Read the job description for the new position. Nothing new to add to my referral. We're revising a document on faculty service to get a new classification. I've seen this before, heard this language before. Create a new letter for Amy, new title. Follow the link in your email. Upload. Submit recommendation. I'm hungry. Turn off the video and just listen. Make a sandwich, toast bread and add mustard. I need to go shopping. Look to make sure I'm muted, they won't hear the chewing. I eat.

"Does that fit with what you were saying Josh?"

I chew quickly, swallow hard, swig coffee. I wipe crumbs from my beard. I haven't shaved in so long. I haven't had a hair cut in so long. I need to get a haircut. I turn on the mic and the video.

"Yea, that makes sense. I agree with what Randy and Paul said. Remove that sentence and it reads better. And then make it 'may' instead of 'should'."

"Thanks, Josh."

Turn off the video. Go on mute again. Finish eating. I should run today. Check email again. Archive. Archive. Delete. Respond to Jasbir. Will it rain? Meeting is over. The election. Talk about how to talk about politics. Talk about doing politics. Setting an example for students. Talk about students. Talk about students doing politics.

"The Mentor": Listen. Post hyperlinks of Michael Silverstein articles on the nation in the Chat box. He's dead now. Post hyperlink to Charles Piot books in the Chat box. Two white guys to start us off. Laughter. Listen. Fire up the Nintendo 64 in your son's room. Start your game and note that you've got almost 70 power stars, which should mean you're close to beating the game. Move Mario so he goes through a door, turns, goes up some stairs, goes through a door, goes up some stairs of the castle, jumps through a portal to an unfinished level. Water and blocks.

Tell the students what you are doing. Call it "wellness gaming" to stay sane during the pandemic. They laugh again. Listen. Play. Listen. Amilcar Cabral insisted on "returning to the source" of non-colonial indigenous life and community.[2] Get a power star from collecting 100 coins (had to beat that robot to get the final five, learned how online last night on YouTube: grab it from behind, hurl it against the wall).

Cabral thought this was necessary in order to search for new possibilities to animate anti-colonial resistance and identification in the present. Get another star by using robots to toss Mario up to the higher platform, then another robot to the next platform (another helpful YouTube tip). Cabral could be a good source for rethinking the nation in Tanzania as a critical Africana theorist. Talk about theory from the south. Feel like you're taking advantage of the students by playing a game with their time along with your own. Think about privilege and exploitation. Stop playing, save your progress, 70 stars now. Talk about method. Talk about theory. Talk about whiteness and blackness and social movements. Talk about names. That person sounds like a Harry Potter character. Strange talking about that now that JK Rowling is a TERF. How do we talk about TERFs? Talk about the Comaroffs. Talk about John Comaraoff now that he's been accused too. How do we talk about people accused of harassment and their work? Talk about talking and writing about politics and not doing politics. Talk about doing politics. Thank everyone. Schedule and make plans.

I sign off. I don't know where to go or what to do. I'm here. I'm here.

Josh Reno

Nine days

Day 1. Friday 30 October

It is the first full day of lockdown. Everything is unfolding quickly: we learned on Wednesday that there would be a second lockdown, the rules were detailed Thursday evening, and the "reconfinement" went into effect Thursday at midnight. The news of lockdown prompts a burst of confusion and movement. My friend who was visiting for the holiday week hurries to return to Paris. Another friend sends a burst of messages:

[10:25 PM, 10/28/2020] You know what?
[10:25 PM, 10/28/2020] We should rent a big house in front of the sea
[10:25 PM, 10/28/2020] And welcome a lot of weird people
[10:25 PM, 10/28/2020] Writers, dancers
[10:26 PM, 10/28/2020] Artist
[10:26 PM, 10/28/2020] I'm sure we could do a great place
[10:26 PM, 10/28/2020] A big house in front of the beach where we would be dancing and writing

Maybe there's an apartment to sublet in my friend's building, at least we would have company. Maybe there's an apartment to housesit while the owners flee to the countryside. Maybe I should just go back to the UK like the University wants us to.

I am packing. After this weekend no travel will be allowed. My fridge is full of food, my laundry hangs damp on the rack, I must scramble.

I check and re-check my "attestation"—the paperwork I must fill out online explaining my motives for travel. I don't know how to use the forms and had to ask a friend. Although we are already in lockdown, the government is tolerating weekend travel so that people can get home from vacation. I am worried about being questioned; I'm not sure I've filled in the right form; I haven't really been on vacation.

As I roll clothes into my suitcase, I notice a car pull up in the street. A woman gets out, then leans in to kiss the driver goodbye. It's past curfew. Is there still a curfew now that we are in lockdown? Well, they are breaking some rule, that seems certain. I note myself noting them. How quickly I absorb the commandments and their enforcement.

Day 2. Saturday 31 October

On the train, I sit pitched forward in my seat, nervous about the attestation. I am returning to an apartment I lived in over the summer, a last-minute solution for the month of reconfinement. When I pull my overloaded suitcase off the train at my old station, I feel visceral relief. After hauling my suitcase up the stairs, I quickly download a second attestation and run to catch the last hour of the weekly market in the main square.

Meandering among the shoppers, I feel elated. I have pulled it off: I have situated myself for lockdown. In celebration, I buy things I have no idea how to prepare like black turnips and prickly pears. I walk by a woman selling seafood, the smell of brine and seaweed. I decide that next week I will figure out how to shuck oysters, and I will eat oysters alone, and I will be happy. I will extract happiness from the lockdown, from this year, like prying an oyster from its shell.

Day 3. Sunday 1 November

I download an attestation to go for a run. Every day, we are allowed one hour of "taking air" within one kilometer of where we live. There's an app that inscribes a circle on a map to show you the permissable boundary. I'd like to walk its circumference, to measure my freedom so precisely.

The park is filled with dog walkers. I have never seen so many people with dogs. Are the dogs being circulated? Is there a service that will deliver you a dog to walk, to take advantage of the dogwalking loophole in the reconfinement rules?

I run along the path by the river in the thick light of evening. I ran this route many times over the summer and began to find it boring, even tedious. But now I feel so lucky that it is within one kilometer of my apartment. I turn off the music, take off my headphones to listen to the river, to the sound of the dry leaves underfoot. The air smells like autumn, like smoke and earth. Freedom can be found in small circles, in familiar places, in interstices.

Day 4. Monday, November 2, 2020

Yesterday, there was an announcement that "non-essential items" will no longer be sold in grocery stores after Tuesday. I immediately ordered an oyster knife on Amazon.

"Don't worry" a friend messages, "this is not a puritanical country, they won't rope off the chocolate and wine aisles." In fact, it is a response to small businesses who have been deemed "non-essential" and have been forced to close complaining that big grocery store chains are nevertheless allowed to sell things books and clothes. On the news, people debate that non-essential closures just drive local business to Amazon.

The US elections loom. In the evening, an attack in Vienna. I literally feel sick to my stomach, but keep watching the news loop. I wake up at 2:00am feeling sick. I am coming down with something. Blowing my nose, I run through the risks I've taken: the train trip, the bathroom in the crowded café, the closed windows in the holiday rental car. I look up "nasal congestion + COVID-19." I get out of bed to see if I can smell things—curry powder and coffee, check, check.

Tomorrow an allergy pill will cure me, but it will take a night of doom-scrolling American politics and COVID symptoms to figure out that it is just the autumn allergies I have every year.

Day 5. Tuesday, November 3, 2020

Election day, Trump ahead. My mom has COVID symptoms. There's an outbreak of a viral mutation among mink in Denmark.

Day 6. Wednesday, November 4, 2020

While half the United States votes for continued authoritarianism and white supremacy, while the country burns, I have work meetings, deadlines, reviews. I feel a bit like when dad died—that strange combination of heartbreak and bureaucracy, that in the midst of being soul-shaken, the paperwork rains down.

Day 7. Thursday 5 November 2020

I spend a lot of time on organizing and arranging things: refolding sheets, placing things just-so on the open shelf in the kitchen, rewriting sentences in emails. Sinking into the smallest details, the drive for control, the aesthetic of anxiety. Today the UK went into lockdown, and my colleagues have a slightly frantic energy. Additional meetings are scheduled. Stay busy. Stay busier.

Day 8. Friday 6 November 2020

The election begins to turn as the ballots are counted. My mom's COVID test comes back negative. I get some cautiously encouraging news about a friend's cancer diagnosis. But I don't trust any of it. A sense of imminent disaster. I wake up and check my phone all night while the rain pours down.

Day 9. Saturday 7 November 2020

I wake up early. I collect my keys and shopping bag, put on my mask, fill out at my attestation—it has become just one more thing in the routine. The market is full of orange autumn fruits and vegetables, squash and persimmon, bright against the gray sky. I buy six oysters and the woman selling them gives me an extra one for "good luck." Just before 5:30 p.m. the election is called for Biden-Harris. I get out my oyster knife.

Alexa Hagerty

Online Lifeline

I am sitting up in bed, typing this on my laptop. It's 11:38PM and I'm wide awake. I periodically check my phone, which is charging from the nightstand to my right (Fig. 2.3).

I've used the service before, not the chat. I had to tell them my gender, that I wasn't trans and what my issues were. After identifying the parking meters to prove I wasn't a robot, I was in. I prefer to call suicide helplines. It feels more personal, I suppose. But I haven't been able to get through the last few times, I suspect it is because of the pandemic. Or the election. Take your pick. "There's nothing wrong with me," I think, "I am wasting their resources. This is fucking stupid." Except a minute ago I was thinking that it would be nice not to be alive again, and this will make me feel better. It has before (Fig. 2.4).

The television is playing an episode from the fourth season of Lost, which I haven't seen in a decade. I don't know why, but about two weeks ago I started rewatching them over again on Amazon Prime from the beginning. Six seasons of people alone with their pain, confused and struggling while stranded on a tropical island. It has an underwhelming ending, I think that is what it is most remembered for. "I should be productive," I think. "Grade, do peer reviewing, schedule meetings, write, reply to emails. I should care more."

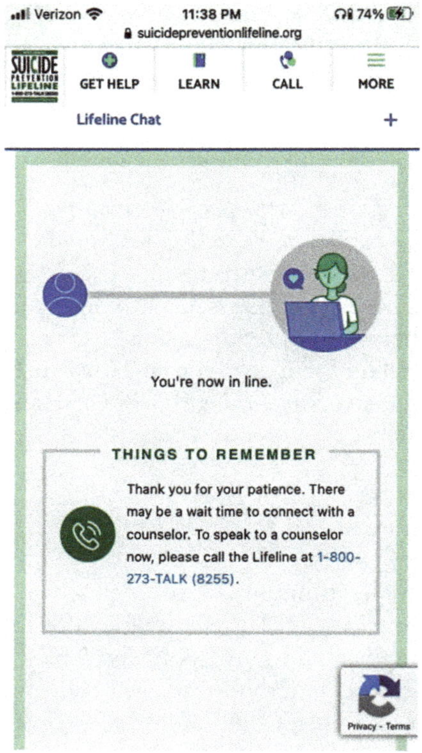

Fig. 2.3 You're now in line. (Photo by J. Reno)

I don't know what I will say, if I ever connect with a counselor. Normally I explain our situation, my son's disability, the challenges of raising him and my history with depression. They say that must be hard on you. They console me and I start to cry. They ask if I have a plan to kill myself, I say not an immediate one, I just don't want to live. They ask are there people I can talk to about this, I pause. One time, the last time I called over a year ago, the woman I spoke with recognized me from calling once before. It was embarrassing but we both laughed.

Sadness is so much like being calm. The fragile heaviness of one's limbs is the same. The lack of impulse, of desire. I especially feel it in my shoulders, my jaw, I don't know why. Maybe it's because my head dips and my face droops. That's what Philippe Bourgois says that heroin addicts do in *Righteous Dopefiend*, they nod, tipping forward barely moving and

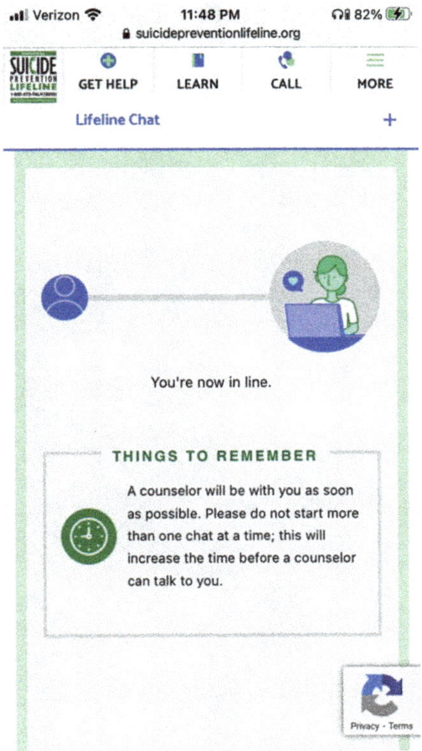

Fig. 2.4 A counselor will be with you soon. (Photo by J. Reno)

drooling in intense pleasure.[3] Sadness addicts like me do the same thing. We nod, heads heavy (Fig. 2.5).

"Am I in a safe space?" My whole life is safe spaces now. I am ensconced in the same small apartment bubble I will eat breakfast in, work in, work out in, nap in, teach in.

I'm not alone right now, not really. My son, Charlie, is rocking in a chair in the living room and humming along to the tv show on his iPad. I don't know why. If I stop staring at the TV and the phone, back and forth and go into the living room, he will leave his chair and abruptly head for another destination. Unlike me, he cultivates alone time, treasures it. His mother is the same, not diagnosed with autism, but a passionate introvert. It's a joke in our house: they would both rather stay home all day and see no one, I would rather go with him to school or with her to the plant and talk to every single person they see every day. Instead I'm stuck here. I go

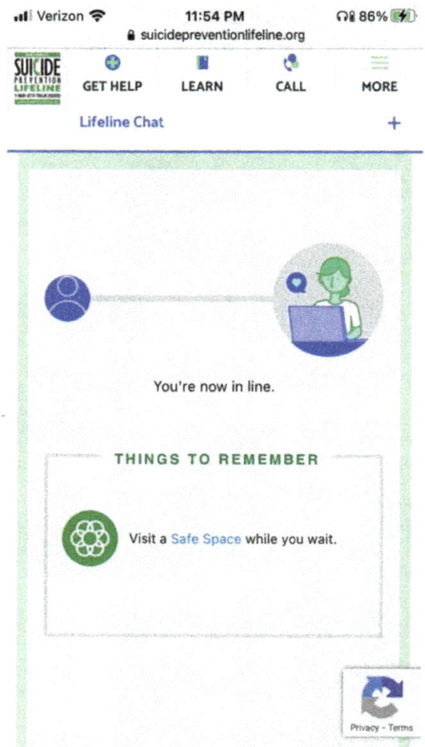

Fig. 2.5 Visit a safe space. (Photo by J. Reno)

nowhere and see no one. It is easier to get sad now, the fix is easier to find. COVID numbers are higher than ever, the election is contested, American health and democracy are on a knife's edge. I just don't want to be alone anymore. I'm so alone. I'm not really alone (Fig. 2.6).

I close the chat. The feelings are gone. It helped to write about them, I guess. Charlie won't stay up too much longer. I'll go to sleep after him, once he gives up and collapses on the bed. I'll stay up after him, all screens turned off, thinking about seeing no one tomorrow, about trying to find a way to care. Eventually, I'll nod off. Tomorrow morning I'll probably feel much better. I don't know why.

Josh Reno

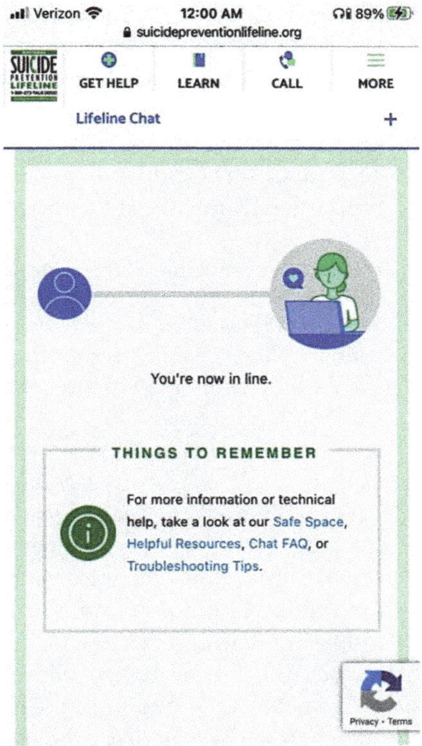

Fig. 2.6 For more. (Photo by J. Reno)

Migrants' Stories in Pandemic Times

I can't sleep peacefully and profoundly anymore. The darkness at night makes my thoughts struggle to quiet down, to fade away, to become dreams, or to just disappear. My thoughts can easily travel across time and space without resting, pausing, or stopping. Our President, not for long, has just announced that whenever a COVID-19 vaccine becomes available in the United States, he won't allow Americans living in New York State to have it. Our Governor reacted with dignity to those remarks. Are those remarks real or is this part of my imagination? Did they really happen? Perhaps I was asleep and this is just part of an ongoing nightmare. My thoughts are racing. Were such gratuitous threats happening also during the past pandemics that humans had to suffer through? I have been reading a lot of stories these days, stories of death and suffering during the

1918-1920 Influenza pandemic, erroneously named "Spanish Flu." Stories that have been re-emerging from books, articles, short essays, and dedicated websites which have resuscitated those dark, forgotten times and places.

While perusing the Internet, I discover, to my surprise, that The Centers for Disease Control and Prevention (CDC) website has a webpage intriguingly entitled "Pandemic Influenza Storybook." Its main description reads:

> The CDC's Pandemic Flu Storybook provides readers with a look at the impact pandemic flu events have had on both survivors and the families and friends of non-survivors. These stories are not folklore, but personal recollections. This collection of stories was first released in 2008 to commemorate the 90th anniversary of the 1918 flu pandemic.[4]

Back in 2008, I didn't even realize it was the 90th anniversary of this deadly pandemic. What was a *pandemic* for many of us in 2008?

I am totally hooked. I spend some of my nights reading as many stories as I can, until my eyes become heavy, until they develop that burning sensation and my vision becomes blurry. An Italian migrant now living in Pennsylvania recounts the story of her Italian grandparents, Nick and Constance, who migrated to the United States during the 1918-1920 flu pandemic. When their seven children caught the virus, Constance had to sleep in a room separated from the one where her children were living and sleeping. To see her children, she had to cover her mouth and nose with a piece of cloth. They had to make cloth masks during that pandemic as well. (The use of masks is not new, in other words.) Four of her children died from the 1918-1920 flu pandemic, two of them were twins. The virus never really interacted with Constance's body. She was lucky. When she was 38, however, she died while she was giving birth to her fourteenth child. Nick, her husband, survived her and died when he was 102. He was never infected by the virus. He made it.

Viruses travel a long way, they cross the ocean, they challenge time and space in unique ways. Four of Nick and Constance's children didn't make it. Their immune system was not strong enough to fight the virus. They didn't have a vaccine available. They didn't have anyone threatening them not to have one. They just died as many other humans did. Their names and moving stories were buried until the CDC decided to make them available on their website in 2008. We too have a virus lingering in the air around us, threatening us, trying to invade our cells to be able to replicate and survive. Yet, we don't seem to learn from past stories such as Constance and Nick's. We commit the same mistakes and hope that we won't be infected. We hope to be lucky. We don't care. We try to defy the coronavirus as many migrants defied the 1918-1920 flu pandemic without even knowing of its existence. That's how history replicates itself in cycles, as Italian philosopher Giambattista Vico long ago taught us.[5]

Sabina M. Perrino

Transnational Pain

A migrant's time is always bracketed. An undocumented migrant's time is always marked by the potential for disruption. An asylum seeker's time is always marked by an indefinite waiting. A stateless person's time is always marked by the lack of a sense of the future.

Throughout the past nine months, it feels like we've been going through cycles of these bracketed temporalities in one form or another. This week, I remarked to students in my seminar on Borders and Mobilities that the pandemic has made us all "feel" what living in these bracketed temporalities can be like. The form that most were able to relate to was that of living in limbo and of endless waiting. Waiting without knowing what's to come, or when the end will be in sight. We were discussing the theme of temporalities as it affects the lives of differently displaced communities and migrants, through readings focused on temporary labor migrants in Israel and undocumented migrants in Southeast Asia. The notions of suspended time, of fragmented family time, of living across multiple time zones, of living without a sense of the future, were all central to our discussions, and it didn't take long for our conversations to take a personal turn when students began realizing just how much of what was being said related to their personal and very immediate experiences.

Students, especially those in more vulnerable situations, experience these pandemic temporalities acutely, in ways that are sometimes impossible for those of us who are privileged to fully understand or empathize with. I can't help but notice the similarities in their stories to those of undocumented migrants and refugees that I used to listen to when we lived in that other world.

My family is no different. We're certainly more privileged and safer than many others, and are fortunate enough to be able to support ourselves and our child through these times. But the pain of being transnational in

COVID times cuts us in so many different ways that still make us feel helpless and powerless. For me, this stretch of suspended time of the pandemic has meant bearing witness to the severe and unbearable suffering of a grandmother who has yet to meet her now one-year-old granddaughter, living halfway across the world. In our home, we have an everyday routine that keeps us occupied, from driving to the daycare, teaching classes, attending endless meetings on Zoom, and doing household errands and chores, while trying to find time to play and entertain each other. There's a comfort in that routine, a sense of time that's reliable and immediate, at least. This mundane temporality is occasionally punctuated by a call or a text message from Malaysia, from a grandmother who longs for photos and videos of the child, who would tell me of her days spent waiting for the next message, photo or video that we send. In those moments, the fragility of the secure tranquility of our mundane temporalities become revealed. I often feel like I'm thrown right back into my childhood home, watching my mother as she occupies her time keeping the house clean, talking on the phone with her sisters, sharing stories of the grandchild she has never met, and spending moments of solitude scrolling through her phone to watch those videos and photos that we send.

That's my experience for the past nine months, but its particular resonance lies in how much it echoes the stories I'd been listening to for so much of my time as an ethnographer of migration and displacement. During times of displacement, disruption, and limbo, it's not the crises or tragedies or other life-changing events that people talk about or obsess over. It's always family and relationships—ones that used to occupy their everyday lives. Most of the migrant women I have met have no interest in talking about their day-to-day lives as domestic helpers, they would always much rather talk about their children and grandchildren back home, in Indonesia, in the Philippines, in Sri Lanka, India, Thailand... they would always be so excited to share their family photos and videos, of children graduating school, of grandchildren taking their first steps... Their time was always elsewhere. In a sense, they rarely saw their own lives in the present of the host country, a space marked by permanent impermanence.

While on the one hand, our current life in the Midwest *feels* full, with the blessing of being able to be so present in the early life of our baby as she grows and discovers her world and herself. But this *fullness* seems to be coupled with that transnational *hollowing* that my parents are experiencing. It feels like as much as we're trying to make the best of our current lives, the reality of grandparents who have been waiting, who continue to wait, and will have to wait without any sense of when they could actually meet their grandchild in person punctuates even the most intimate and sweetest of moments. Our daughter's first birthday, which we organized over Skype with grandparents in Italy and Malaysia, was painfully bitter-sweet, as was seeing the little one try to stand and take her first steps the past two weeks. We're somewhat fortunate in that as a couple we're both able to relate and share this experience of being transnational immigrants, for which I'm thankful.

But what about the countless others around the world who are being forced to wait indefinitely, watching life and the lives of their distant loved ones, pass them by so quickly?

Parthiban Muniandy

Breathing with Others

Behind a half-open garage-door is my neighborhood gym, which I went back to six months after it temporarily shut down in March 2020.

I stepped inside, and I saw about half a dozen people wearing masks with various colors and shapes. Next to the rectangles where people work out, and I noticed two big, towering air filters with a shining green light, presumably indicating that the filter is still brand-new.

Good ventilation and air filters, I thought, I can breathe safely in here.

Fred, who works at the front desk, greeted me, and waved his hand. A student at a nearby college, his cheery disposition stood in contrast to the serious facial expressions that some people make when they are about to attempt a heavy deadlift. Fred held a small thermometer, and I showed him my left wrist. 96.3 degrees, it showed.

"You're good to go!" he said.

Funny, it could be just the fact that I was standing outside in the cold wind. That's why, I thought, I'm always stone cold at these temperature checks.

This local gym is perhaps the only other part of my life that involves interacting with others in person other than the grocery store or the drug store. It is as if the only thing that requires interacting in person is the need to maintain my physical health. I enjoy going here, though, because it is a contrast to the absolute lack of physical exercise that I experienced during my dissertation fieldwork.

My mind wandered. Why is it, I thought, that ethnographers are often expected to speak through the experiences of their mind, and not of their bodies? Although my scholarly career is shaped primarily through paperwork and computer files, I also experience working as an anthropologist through the aches, soreness, and fatigues that I experienced before, during, and after fieldwork.

My mind traveled back to the gym. I looked at the rig in front of me, and I wonder if I could do pull-ups, which I struggled to do even before the pandemic.

I did my warm-ups, and I looked at others around me: are they wearing their masks properly? Should I choose another spot on the gym floor where I am a bit farther away from others?

Ben, the coach, gave us instructions on how to accomplish a tricky movement, the kettlebell thruster. This was part of a workout that also involved burpees [squat-thrusts], so, unsurprisingly, everyone's heart rates went way up, mine too. It was a combination of being out of breath while making sure that I hold a proper grip on the kettlebell, an oddly shaped weight, so that it does not hurt my wrists.

I checked my digital watch—my heart rate is at 182, and I was almost out of breath.

I looked around me, and I saw others peeking through their masks to catch a breath. Others quickly sipped some water while trying to ensure that their face masks cover both their mouths and the water bottle.

I thought to myself, well, the risks for contracting a contagious virus here are not exactly zero either.

"Guys!" said Ben, quite forcefully. "If you want this gym to stay open, please keep your masks on! I don't fuck around with that!"

We all looked at Ben, who did not seem very pleased.

As I grabbed the kettlebell, trying to make sure that it does not hit my wrists again, I thought that the risks for contracting this virus here is not zero. It is perhaps a substantial risk.

After the workout ended, I laid down on the floor to wait for my heart rate to go down

"Good job guys! Don't forget to wipe everything after you're done!" said Ben.

What a strange time, I thought—how could human breath be thought of as pollutants, matters out of place in a world full of many other breathing beings?

My breathing and my heart rate gradually went back to normal, and I started cleaning the surfaces around me with a disinfecting wipe. I was glad that, for now, I can breathe freely.

Rafadi Hakim

The Paranoid Style

He works out, that's clear from the tight t-shirt. He has tested positive for COVID-19, but—and this is key—he suffers no symptoms.

The president's son, Don Jr., is quarantined in a cabin. I hear the news on BBC radio. In my imagination it is snowing, and he is feverish, but he denies he is ill and insists on hunting. I imagine him staggering through the snow, hallucinating and weak, in some recasting of a Jack London story I vaguely remember from elementary school about hubristic masculinities and death in the wilderness.

I do a quick google search and land on a video Don Jr. has posted on Instagram.[6] He is standing in a self-consciously rustic cabin with hunting trophies on the wall--*aha*, I think, *I was right about the hunting*! Don Jr. tells the camera, "Apparently I got the 'rona'." He rambles. He could be feverish, I think. He says he was supposed to go on a trip with his son. "Gotta cancel that trip," he says. Unbidden, I feel sorry for him. I have never imagined him as a father, but only as an unloved son, desperately seeking approval. He says, "I may have a couple days of solo time and there's only so many guns I can clean before that gets bored [sic]."

Fathers, sons, and guns. It all seems to fit together.

Don Jr.'s t-shirt says EBERLESTOCK. I google the brand and find it is outdoor gear designed by a "veteran, Olympian, and dedicated backcountry hunter." A Guardian article says, "Trump Jr is believed to have political ambitions beyond being just his father's son and has successfully courted popularity with the Republican party's conservative base, carefully cultivating an outdoorsy and hunting popular image" (Guardian). The shirt, the cabin, the guns, it all seem carefully chosen. Like a stage set. Like a clue to something.

Richard Hofstadter's famous article "The Paranoid Style in American Politics" was first published in Harper's Magazine, November 1964.[7] Eve Kosofsky Sedgwick theorized a crucial development, that Hofstadter's vision of paranoia, albeit widespread, nevertheless contained "a presumptive 'we'—apparently still practically everyone—that can agree to view such extremes from a calm, understanding, and encompassing middle ground." This "we" has vanished, if it ever existed at all; paranoid thinking has become normative across the political spectrum. "In a funny way," writes Sedgwick, "I feel closer today to … [the paranoid] than I do to Hofstadter."[8]

I google "Don Jr." + "hunting." A clickbait headline announces: "President Donald Trump's two adult sons Eric and Donald Trump, Jr. own a huge, private hunting range in a rural community in upstate New York. Neighbors report hearing massive explosions and shooting from the property. The property is located next to an abandoned psychiatric hospital that is said to be haunted." The land abuts the old potter's field. Haunted psychiatric hospital? Oh yes, *Business Insider*, I will scroll onward.

The article tells me that when the Trumps bought the property, they "tried to reduce the price by invoking a 1991 state court decision that requires buyers disclose to sellers if a property is known to be haunted." Part of me thinks this is very Scooby-doo, and part of me thinks of the people instutionalized once in the old state hospital, and what they suffered, and what the most vulnerable among us will continue to suffer as the mad king guts our health systems and social safety nets. The dead have their reasons for haunting.

I keep googling. A *ProPublica* article tells me that in 2019 Don Jr. hunted and killed an endangered argali sheep in Mongolia. I think of the hunting trophies in Don Jr.'s Instagram. I take a screenshot of a skull mounted on the wall and zoom in.

In an article exploring the welter of "frauds, leaks, lies, paranoiac mass movements, and imagined conspiracies" that mark American political history, a scholar urges us to understand "the affective—even libidinal—aesthetic qualities of the conspiracy theory."[9] In other words, it is not in careful analysis and cool-headed theory that conspiracy most clearly reveals itself, but through its strange pleasures.

I toggle back and forth between tabs, between hunting trophies and photos of argali sheep. Examining the grainy screenshot, I decide it isn't an endangered species. Is that a price tag dangling from the horn? I wonder why they have chosen these hunting trophies as props, what it means. I google "goat's skull significance." This is a mistake. My top results:

www.quora.com › Is-a-goat-skull-a-sign-of-satanism
Dec 30, 2016—A goat skull is not a sign of Satanism; it is only a sign of a dead goat

Baphomet—Wikipediaen.wikipedia.org › wiki › Baphomet
[...] Sigil of Baphomet · Éliphas Lévi · Trials of the Knights Templar · Horned deity

This is not really a rabbit hole I want to go down. I feel vaguely creeped out from reading about satanism and also kind of dirty because I have spent my Sunday morning stalking Don Jr., searching for clues to something (what exactly?). Feeling prurient and guilty, I close the tabs. I notice that in the screenshot of Don Jr's cabin, just under the ram's skull, there is a teddy bear hanging from the wall. It is like a punchline to a joke: my paranoid searching has led to this absurd dead end. The wrongs of this moment in history, the deep political sins of this time are not hidden. I don't have to zoom in on grainy images. It is all out in the open, happening right in front of us (Fig. 2.7).

Alexa Hagerty

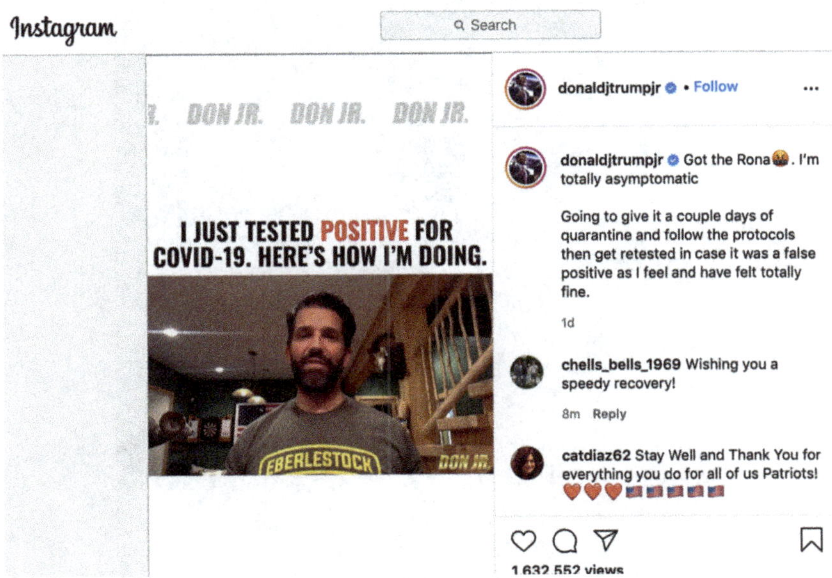

Fig. 2.7 Screen capture of Donald Trump Jr.'s Instagram page November 21, 2020

Goldilocks-Down

Lockdown Day #XX?

I sit on my wooden chair by the window. Get some sunshine, I tell myself. Make some tea, grab a blanket, go outside. I head into the garden—how lucky I am to have one during the second lockdown. Voices from the apartments above filter down. I test my limits: leaning back and balancing on the two legs of this plastic chair for as long as I can, dreaming of filling the three other cracked chairs with friends (Fig. 2.8).

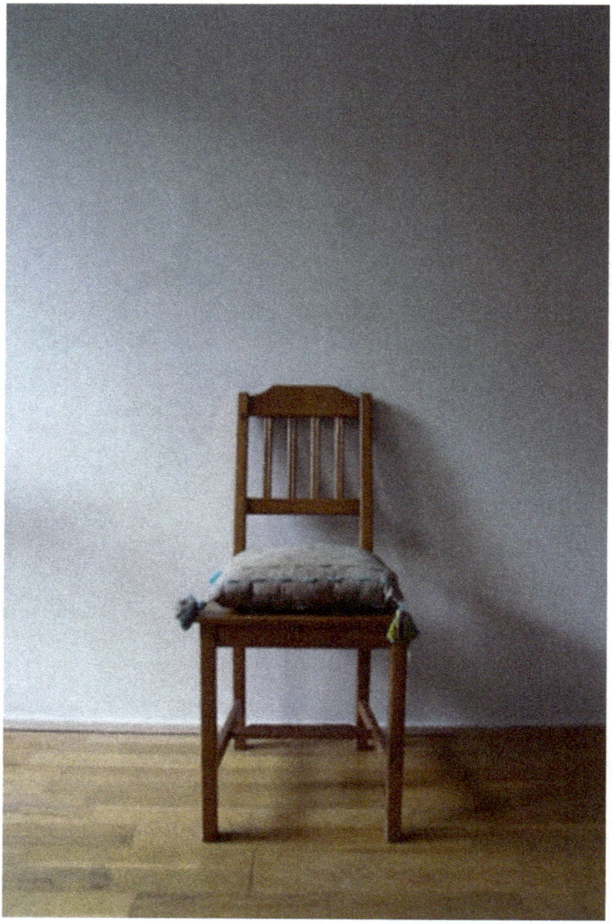

Fig. 2.8 A Wooden Chair. (Photo by M. Fitoussi)

Thirty minutes later, I move inside to the wicker chair. I last twenty minutes; damn, this chair really doesn't work for me, its long, narrow back pressing into my spine. Next, the ceramic chair, yes, the toilet. The bathroom is sacred, the place I used to sit and do my math homework after a hot shower and a three-hour swim practice. Something about the humidity and the fact that I could lock the door, the only solitude in a noisy, crowded house. But I don't last long in this lonely bathroom. Back to my wooden chair. In fact, there are three wooden chairs situated around the table—seemingly identical. I try out the other two. The first is rickety, the second—I can't quite name it, something is off about the angle of its back. I think about the people who bought proper desk chairs at the start of the pandemic. I return to my wooden chair. Cross my legs, add a pillow, sit on its edge, rock on the back legs. *Avoid the futon bed at all costs.*

It's now 7:00 p.m., curfew in two hours. I leave the house in the dark: 1 kilometer, 1 hour, with an attestation, a sort of laissez-passer, that you sign and date—a document where you write your address, your place of birth (why?), and tick the box justifying why you are leaving your house. I walk more than an hour, I walk outside the 1 km radius, I reuse an attestation from yesterday. I want to see my brother tonight but he's hesitant to break curfew.

I put more and more distance between myself and my apartment. I walk the empty, hilly streets of Belleville wondering what makes a place a home, my home. Crown Heights, Harlem, Morningside Heights, Somerville, Cambridge, Tunis, Seal Beach, Obo, Kampala, Dungu, Berkeley, Cape Town, Long Beach, Paris. What makes a place home? Coffee made the same way. A sheer dress hung on the wall. A blanket arranged loosely on the bed. A wooden chair by the window.[10]

Margaux Fitoussi

Chronochromatic Maps

I look at the screen: mesmerizing viral maps populate our mediascapes. Europe is tinted with different hues of red, yellow, and orange (Figs. 2.9 and 2.11).

The US electoral map is instead drastically divided between red states and blue states (Fig. 2.10). Time seems to flow at a slower pace as I try to focus and diffuse the anxiety that envelops these early November days. I look at the maps in search of solace from the grip of the blurred temporality of suspense. The colors change as time goes by, indicating the shifts in

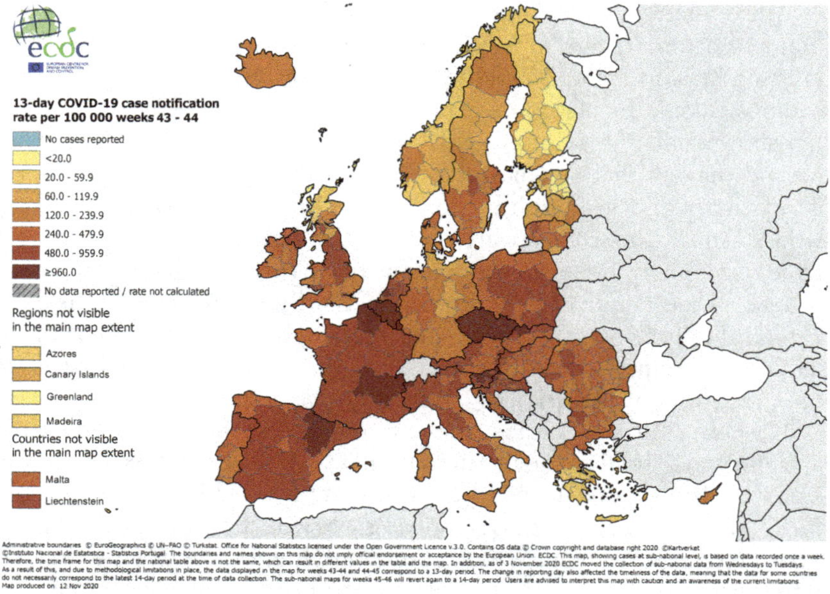

Fig. 2.9 A map produced on November 12, 2020, indicating the rate of COVID-19 Notifications recorded within the European Union between October 19 and November 1, 2020. Courtesy of ©ECDC [2005–2022]

the ballot count in the US and the progression of the contagion in Europe. Two political and sanitary cartographies gesturing at two different types of suspension and uncertainty: the unpredictable results of the US presidential race and the unfathomable consequences of the inevitable spread of the virus.

Here we go again, the second wave has begun. Its grip over Europe is now apparent. The summer lull has given way to a new season of infections. Virus talk has replaced small weather chatter as a new form of phatic communion.

"My hope is that the virus will go away in the summer and never come back because of the heat, just like SARS did," wrote a friend and colleague based in Vienna, back in April. At times, during the Mediterranean summer, I too entertained the fleeting illusion that the pandemic was behind us. After a long winter spent in the desolate realm of daily bulletins of confirmed and projected cases, death tolls, and contagion indexes, with the summer breeze, the bombardment of numbers and statistical data momentarily stopped. The techno-rationality of quantification and

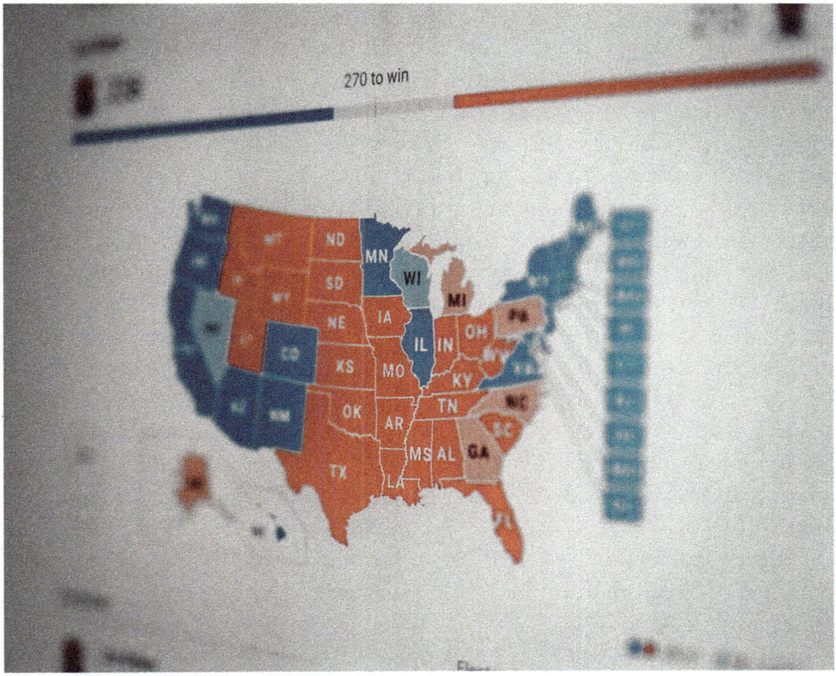

Fig. 2.10 A chromopolitical map of the US Presidential race, November 4, 2020. Courtesy of Clay Banks, on Unsplash

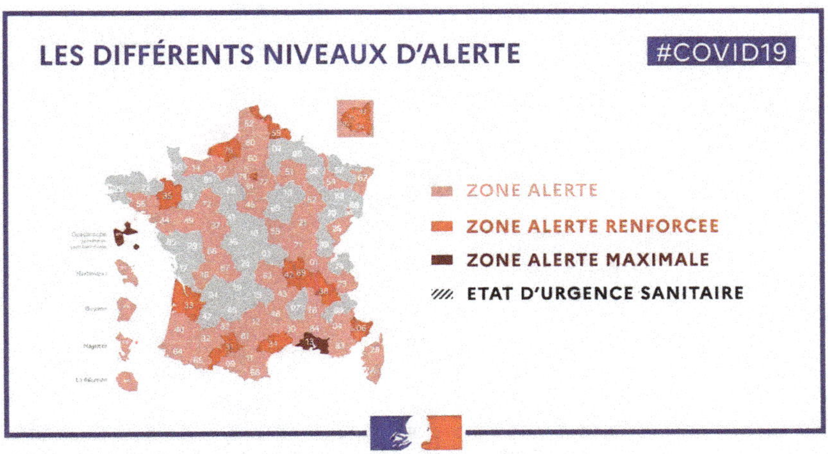

Fig. 2.11 Different alert levels in France as of September 23, 2020. Map by Ministre des Solidarités et de la Santé, the French Ministry of Health

predictive analytics gave way to ephemeral flashes of hope and radical uncertainty: "maybe it won't come back, maybe it'll disappear, mysteriously, like SARS did." As Arjun Appadurai would put it, the future appeared again as a horizon of possibilities unregimented by the stringent logic of probability calculation.[11] A short-lived illusion ushered away by the new viral season. "The French have 50,000 a day!" say people in Italy with a mixture of astonishment and condescending hubris, pretending to ignore the memories of the first wave and indulging themselves in the illusion that time could be somehow frozen, so that they will not follow suit. But in our new pandemic lifeworld, the elsewhere is but a preemptive figuration of our own foreseeable future. The temporal logic of the contagion's exponential progression is now again redesigning the cartography of our daily lives. Paris and the Ile-de-France region were declared red zones at the beginning of the fall. A new map of France was released on September 24, 2020, marking with varied shades of red the different levels of hazard and different degrees of restrictions enforced in each region (Fig. 2.11).[12]

The perimeters of risk and fear entertain an awkward overlap with national and regional boundaries, regulating norms of conduct as well as collective affects.

At the beginning of November, Italy was split into three color-coded zones associated with different regimes of restrictions: red (high-risk), orange (medium-risk), and yellow (low-risk). As we gradually but inexorably go back into a lockdown mode, these new chronochromatic maps, with their temporally shifting color-codes (Fig. 2.12), redesign the

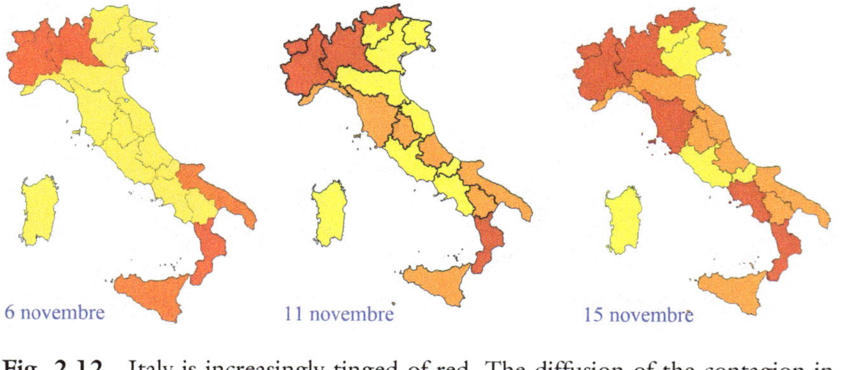

Fig. 2.12 Italy is increasingly tinged of red. The diffusion of the contagion in the span of nine days. (November 6 to November 15, 2020). (Courtesy of AMnotizie)

perimeters of our progressively circumscribed existences—setting novel boundaries to our imaginations, temporalities, and whereabouts.[13]

Aurora Donzelli

Alone, Performing to the Wall

I was feeling antsy. Though I'd moved two seminars online in the Spring, one of my Fall courses was a lecture with 120 enrolled students. That size for an online class felt daunting. I had taught various iterations of this course, which focused on mental health and healing in East Asia, several times before. My hope was this "meat and potatoes" offering would be amenable to a pandemic re-heating.

In the days leading up to the first day of classes, I kept trying different configurations in my office. Sitting didn't feel appropriate to face a class of that size. I eventually settled on standing behind a homemade podium created by wedging a wicker table on top of a chair, and spoke at an external camera I positioned on my bookshelf. Less than five minutes before the first class, I was fiddling with the camera when I heard a crash behind me. A mounted painting had fallen to the floor, cracking its heavy frame and leaving a hole in the wall.

Despite my misgivings, the initial meetings felt OK. As the weeks past, however, I began to dread talking to the bookshelf. Part of the problem was the profound disconnection I felt from the students. The great majority of those attending turned their cameras off for most of the class, leaving me facing a sea of black squares on my zoom screen. I could, however, catch the *number* of students that I was speaking to. This figure decreased throughout the semester, from 90s in the first weeks into the 70s, 60s, 50s. While my comments were recorded and posted, the sagging viewing numbers led me to feel a corresponding quantity of energy was seeping out of our virtual classroom. I tried engaging students by increasing my use of polls and breakout rooms, modifying assignments, writing out more of my lectures. Nothing seemed to help.

The most disturbing part of the experience was the way that performing in front of the camera seemed to be affecting my thinking. I had always prepared for courses by printing out a couple of pages of notes and then generally ignoring them, my thoughts coming together, more or less, in the moment. In recent weeks, I found myself feeling dully and fuzzy during class, unable to predict if I would be able to offer coherent thoughts.

Last Tuesday, the murkiness got worse. The assigned text was Claude Lévi-Strauss's essay on the effectiveness of symbols. The piece has long been a favorite of mine. The symbolic function of the unconscious, aided by collective (although also potentially personal) myth, allows the Cuna shaman to perform a "cure" precipitating his sick pregnant patient to return to "an order which is no longer threatened" where "conflicts and resistances are resolved."[14] I find the overly neat structuralist world with its bold vision of the human mind, creative parallelisms, and most of all decisive presentation of the cure to be reassuring. Yet my own inability to effectively explain the material left me in a panic that lingered after the lecture ended. I began to wonder if it might possible to cancel classes or find some way to escape from what was left of the semester. I didn't want to go in front of the camera again.

While still in a funk the next morning, I had the opportunity to speak with individuals enrolled in the class during office hours. In particular, two students in separate appointments shared how they were anxious, distracted, barely getting by, struggling to finish the semester. The honest conversations were deeply helpful to me as I could finally feel how emotions that were increasingly overwhelming me were shared by others.

The brief encounters were certainly no cure: my conflicts and resistances, in particular towards the hated camera on the wall, continue. But those Zoom meetings were enough to convince me that it was possible for us to muddle our way through the last part of the semester.

Nicholas Bartlett

Fresh Flowers and State Violence

The year 2020 is drawing to an end, but its uncanny imagery still lingers over Milan during the New Year's Eve lockdown. Novel vistas of expansive empty urban spaces have saturated our vision during the pandemic, leaving us in breathless contemplation of the spectral spectacle of what the world looks like in the aftermath of humanity. As I walk through Piazza Fontana with an auto-certification in my pocket (stating that I am not infected with COVID-19, that I have valid reasons to leave my domicile and that I am aware of the criminal sanctions for making false statements), I feel dazed. Unlike the usual bustle, a strange stillness enwraps this small square lying behind the city's main cathedral. I dawdle like an unseen spirit, walking past the site where, on December 12, 1969, a terrorist bombing left 17 dismembered corpses on the ground. Although the attack was carried out by neo-fascist groups and masterminded by deviated secret services, the blame was placed on left-wing militants and anarchists. I notice the fresh flowers a human hand placed next to the stone plaque commemorating Giuseppe Pinelli *railroad worker and anarchist innocently killed in Milan's central police station on December 15, 1969.* A few days ago, an interview

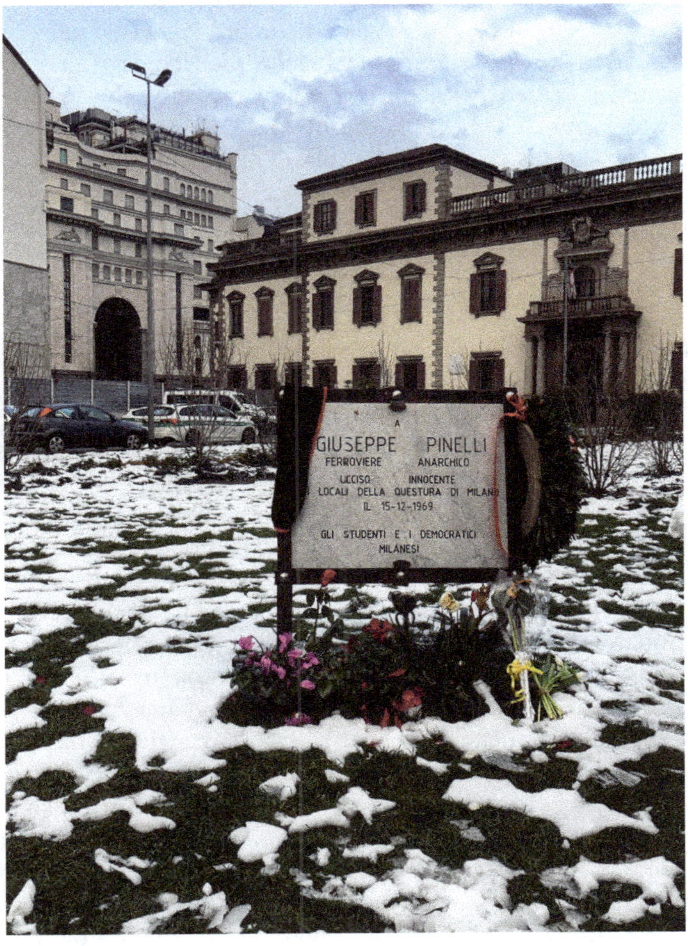
A
GIUSEPPE PINELLI
FERROVIERE ANARCHICO
UCCISO INNOCENTE
LOCALI DELLA QUESTURA DI MILANO
IL 15-12-1969
GLI STUDENTI E I DEMOCRATICI
MILANESI

Piazza Fontana, Milan. The stone plaque placed "by the student and the democrats of Milan" commemorating Giuseppe Pinelli. (Photo by A. **Donzelli)**

with the then second in command of Italy's intelligence agency (SID), General Gianadelio Maletti, finally shed light on how Pinelli was killed during a brutal police interrogation: "Pinelli would refuse to answer questions or gave irritating answers. The interrogators therefore resorted to stronger means and threatened to throw him out of the window if he persisted in staying silent. They forced him to sit on the window ledge. With each negative response, Pinelli was pushed a little more towards the void. Until he finally lost his balance and fell."[15] Fifty-one years ago, Pinelli was pushed into the void for a crime he had not committed after being illegally held in custody for three days. Today, an empty Piazza Fontana reverberates with ghostly presences of state violence: the victims of the Italy's first major state massacre, the victims of police brutality, the victims of the profit-driven approach to public health that killed thousands of elderly residents in the city's care homes.[16] Still no justice, just fresh flowers.

Aurora Donzelli

Deferred Returns

The latest beginning of the end of pandemic restrictions is underway. In mid-May, I had my first coffee in a café, and, a couple days later, my first meal in an unequivocally "indoor" restaurant. Barnard College, my employer, announced there will not be social distancing restrictions in the classrooms this fall. New York is back in business, the politicians say.

With teaching over, my attention in recent weeks has turned elsewhere: I have a year of leave to start a new research project, and have been planning to move to Asia. I have been invited to participate in a conference exploring unconscious group dynamics scheduled to take place in Wuhan. I'm unsure if the Chinese authorities will allow the conference to meet in person, or if I will be able to get into the country to attend. Several months ago, I submitted applications to potential hosts in mainland China. They have remained in a queue, unprocessed. More recently, I started making contacts in Taiwan. An outbreak there this month has introduced additional uncertainties to this back-up plan. The family calendar is empty after July, but it is far from certain if and when will be able to travel. The message from all contacts across the Pacific is the same: "Wait and see."

This uncertainty has changed the way that I follow news and track casual conversations. I find myself collecting and returning to the stories of friends and colleagues who have become stuck, who are waiting, watching, hoping to be able to move to see partners and family members or start new learning and work opportunities. A student and I commiserate on Zoom; he is in Shanghai and doesn't know if he will be able to get back to New York in the fall. A one-way plane ticket for the day he wants to return is $10,000 and the US embassy and consulates have been canceling visa appointments at the last minute. His classmates quarantine in Bangkok, Singapore, or the Middle East on their way back to New York. Meanwhile, new outbreaks in Morocco, Argentina, and India increase anxiety about the spread of new variants. Despite my own better judgment, I also begin to closely monitor infection and vaccine figures in the region. After a slow start, the People's Republic has been averaging more than 20 million shots a day, 100 million people in a week.

In mid-May, the publication of an open letter in *Science* magazine from a group of experts has attracted new interest to the Wuhan "lab-leak hypothesis" and the role of human error in the spread of COVID-19. I do not like the accusatory language or the self-righteousness of those who see an opportunity to attack the People's Republic in a moment when closer collaboration is desperately needed. Part of my reaction undoubtedly comes from my own selfish wish to avoid exacerbating the growing rift between the People's Republic and the US, a rift that potentially impacts my family's impending move.

New details from the origins controversy discussions resonate with my own pre-pandemic history in China in unexpected ways. The abandoned copper mine where the alleged COVID-precursor was excreted in bat droppings is located in the southern part of Yunnan, less than 80 miles from Gejiu, the mining community where I conducted my dissertation research. I know people who were involved in copper mining, potentially who had even worked in those mountains. Moreover, the event of interest—a mysterious pneumonia outbreak that caused the death of three workers cleaning guano from the cave—occurred in 2012 when I was nearby.

A couple of night ago, I had a dream: I am back in Gejiu at last, happy to be wandering the city's streets and meeting up with old friends. But in the middle of my visit, foreign planes arrive and bomb the city. I shout out to nearby residents that buildings are on fire as I run for the safety of the lake at the center of the city.

In the end, I don't know what is coming. I still hope to be able to travel with my family to Taiwan, to mainland China, and, especially, to southern Yunnan. In my initial reflections, this desire persisted in spite of virus-related barriers, but now my wish to return seems entangled with the pandemic in ways I struggle to understand. So much remains uncertain. There is nothing to do but wait.

Nicholas Bartlett

Notes

1. Moten (2017: 219).
2. Cabral (1973).
3. Bourgois (2009).
4. https://www.cdc.gov/publications/panflu/index.html
5. Vico (1725).
6. https://www.instagram.com/p/CH1c_h8A7AI/
7. Hofstadter (1964).
8. Sedgwick (2003).
9. Fraser (2020).
10. In order to illustrate the notion of structure, Roland Barthes invokes the image of the ship *Argo*. In the myth of Jason and the Argonauts, the Greek Gods ordered them to carry out the entire journey in the same ship, the Argo, with the knowledge that it would very likely fall apart. The parts of the entire ship were replaced over the course of the journey, but it remained the same in *name* and in *form*. This, for Barthes, revealed how the "system prevails over the very being of objects" (1994, 46).
11. Appadurai (2013).
12. On October 25 2020, France registered a record 52,010 new confirmed coronavirus per day and went into a second lockdown on October 30.
13. https://www.amnotizie.it/2020/11/14/litalia-si-tinge-sempre-piu-di-rosso-ed-arancione-restano-solo-5-aree-in-zona-gialla/ (last accessed, April 3, 2022).
14. Lévi-Strauss, Claude. "The Effectiveness of Symbols." Structural anthropology, translated by Clair Jacobson and Brooke Grundfest Schope. New York: Basic Books, 1963.
15. *Il Fatto quotidiano*, December 11, 2020, "Misero Pinelli sul davanzale. Fu così che poi cadde e morì" by Alberto Nerazzini e Andrea Sceresini. https://www.ilfattoquotidiano.it/in-edicola/articoli/2020/12/11/misero-pinelli-sul-davanzale-fu-cosi-che-poi-cadde-e-mori/6033384/ (last accessed, April 3, 2022).
16. For more details on the violations of the human rights of older residents of care homes in Lombardy during the COVID-19 pandemic, see the recent report by Amnesty International https://www.amnesty.org/en/latest/news/2020/12/italyviolations-of-the-h-uman-rights-of-older-residents-of-care-homes-during-COVID-19-pandemic/ (last accessed, April 3, 2022). For an account of Italy's Strategy of Tension and State Massacres, see the recent book by Enrico Deaglio (2019).

CHAPTER 3

Part III: Photos from the New Year

The idea now is for all of us to submit a photograph or two around the New Year, with the images reflecting the author's thoughts on the year that has passed (2020), as well as the year to come (2021). A brief text should accompany the images, anything from a sentence or two to a paragraph. The images can be drawn from any time, but the writing should be composed around the New Year. As one of us wrote recently, "It just seems that '2020' has become such a signifier of all that has happened, and thus has a magnetic affective field around it, and this could be a way to capture the sense of movement of time and periodization within our collection, which also mirrors the movements of global yet-dispersed collective experience to a certain degree..."
December 2020

R. Desjarlais et al., *Dispatches from Home and the Field during the COVID-19 Pandemic*, Palgrave Studies in Literary Anthropology,
https://doi.org/10.1007/978-3-031-19193-0_3

CHANGE (FIGS. 3.1 AND 3.2)

Emily Ng

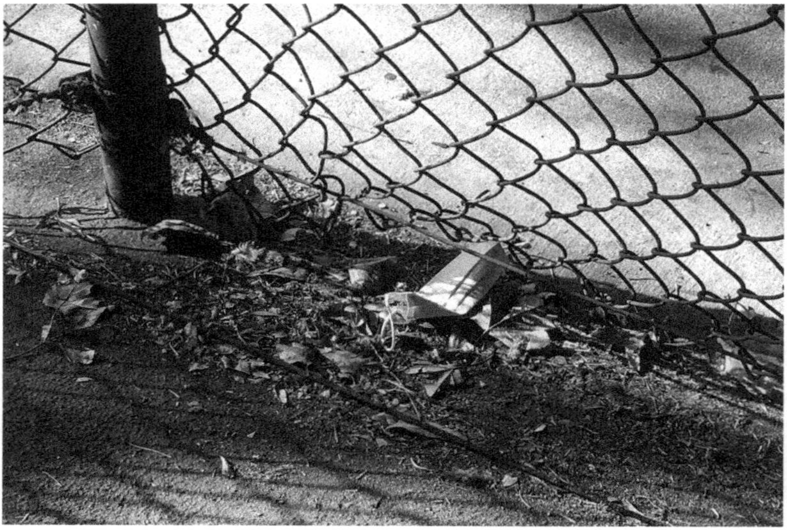

Fig. 3.1 Oakland, California. December 2020. (Photo by E. Ng)

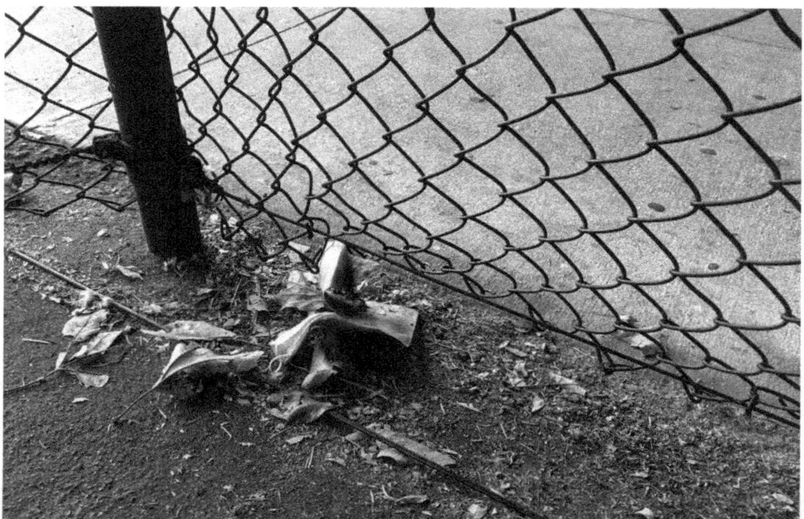

Fig. 3.2 Oakland, California. January 2021. (Photo by E. Ng)

Boy, It's Scary Out There

In one of the great film series of the twentieth century, ten-year-old Kevin McCallister runs furiously through Central Park and jumps into the back of a taxi. He says to the cab driver, "Boy, it's scary out there!" The driver turns around slowly with his Frankenstein-ish face and growls, "Ain't much better in here kid." McCallister screams and runs back out into the void.

A philosophical exchange worthy of 2020 (Fig. 3.3).

Maybe, just maybe, 2021 will be better (Fig. 3.4).

Margaux Fitoussi
January 2021

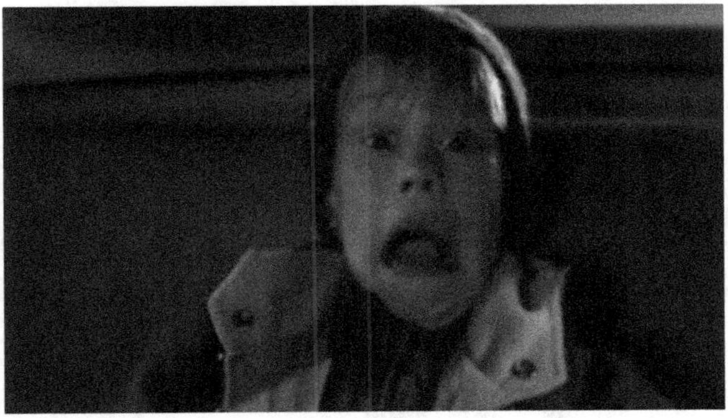

Fig. 3.3 A screenshot from *Home Alone 2*

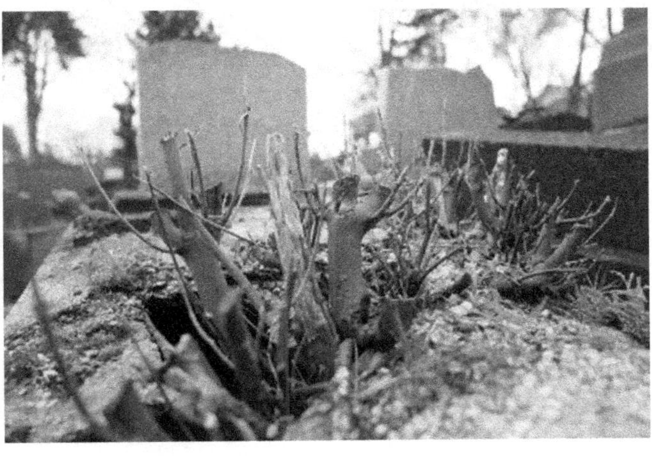

Fig. 3.4 Belleville Cemetery, Paris. (Photo by M. Fitoussi)

The Same River Twice (Fig. 3.5)

The same river twice. The river does not change from the old year to the new. But it changes from hour to hour. Day after day, you get better at seeing it. Hold on. Hold onto the earth and its changes. The evening light lasted longer today.

Alexa Hagerty
January 2021

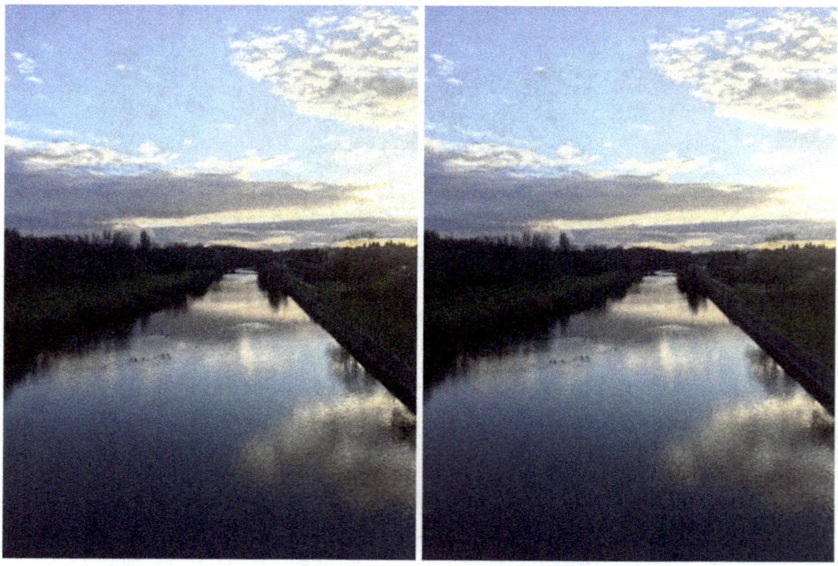

Fig. 3.5 The Aude River. (Photo by A. Hagerty)

A Sign of the Times (Fig. 3.6)

The sign caught my eye on New Year's Eve, while I was driving on a road that connects Yonkers to Bronxville, in the suburban metropolis of Westchester County, New York. The green and yellow placard is set at the entrance to a small woodlands park that runs along the Bronxville River, near to the Bronx River Expressway. The reminder to practice safe social distancing is a commonplace, commonsensical statement these days. Take care not to spread the virus. Yet in contemplating the sign while at a nearby intersection, waiting for the light to turn green, I gave thought to the fact that if the same sign had been placed in this same location precisely a year ago, before the pandemic hit, few would have known what it could possibly mean or stand for. I might have read the words as an odd New Year's Eve jest, or as a clue leading to a clandestine riverbank party playfully arranged by local teenagers. And perhaps, in a year's time, or two, the sign will have been rendered obsolete, a discarded image of past troubles. Our language has taken on new qualities and significations, as has our

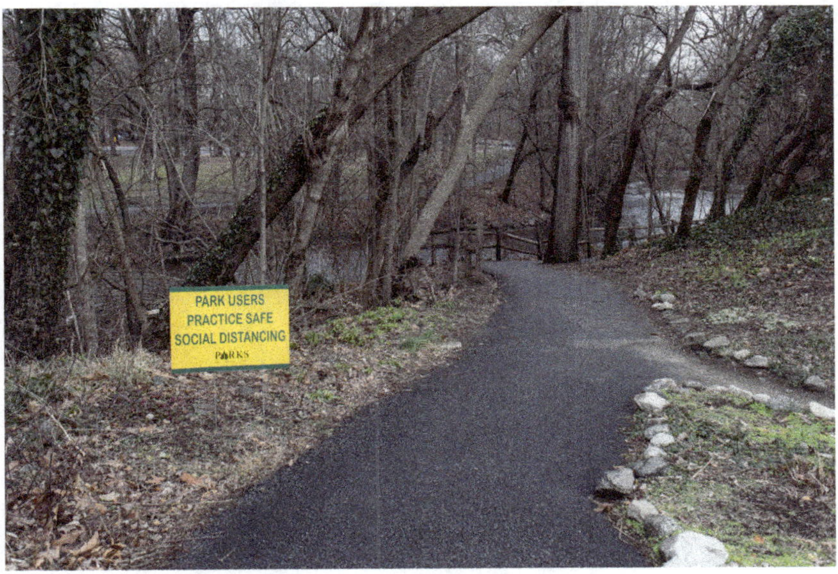

Fig. 3.6 Park by a stretch of the Bronx River, Bronxville, New York. January 1, 2021. (Photo by R. Desjarlais)

experience of the world. “What, in the end, makes advertisements so superior to criticism?” Walter Benjamin wrote in *Two-Way Street*. “Not what the moving red neon sign says — but the fiery pool reflecting it in the asphalt.”[1] Chances are that, if encountering this sign, anyone who has lived through the plague year of 2020 would be able to pick up on the muddy, miasmic densities reflected in the asphalt sidewalk, and the river below.

Robert Desjarlais

Photo of a Photo (Fig. 3.7)

This is a photograph of a photograph, a way of documenting the past that I found increasingly common as printed photographs gave way to digital photography. Lacking the time and the motivation to reproduce old family photos, I took pictures of them using my phone, and shared these images—decades after my grandmother and great-aunt, pictured, here, smiled at the camera.

At a time when in-person visits and family reunions are suspended, these images, sent over text messages and social media, make shared moments of remembrance possible.

Although this particular photo was taken in Jakarta by a family friend sometime in 1988, I took this picture-of-a-picture almost thirty years later, in 2016. In the summer of 2016, while browsing through a photo album, I captured this image using my phone, because the photo showed

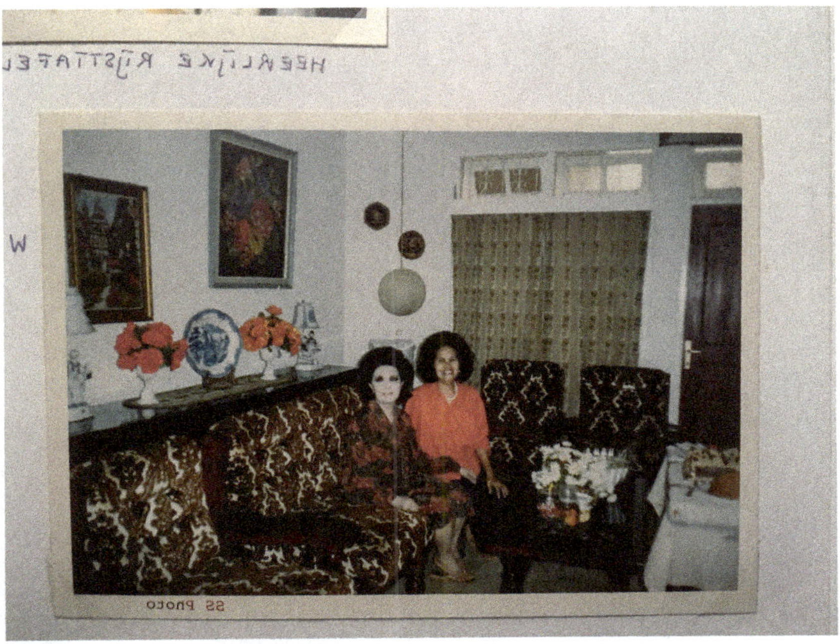

Fig. 3.7 Photo of a photo of Bebi (left) and Wien (right) in Jakarta, Indonesia, around 1988. (Photo by R. Hakim)

two individuals whom I remember fondly: my grandmother, Wien, who died in 1999, and her younger sister, Bebi, who died recently, in September 2020.

For four years, this photo stayed in my phone's cloud storage, untouched and unshared with others, until September 2020, right after Bebi's death, when I wanted to find a way to remember both her and my own grandmother. In the middle of pandemic-related travel restrictions, I could not attend her funeral in Jakarta, which is thousands of miles away from Chicago, where I live. Nevertheless, I decided to remember the two sisters in a different way: I uploaded this photo to my Facebook profile, and I wrote about how the two sisters were reunited after more than two decades apart.

As 2020 came to a close, I tried to find a picture that represented my experiences during the year of the pandemic, and I stopped the moment this image appeared on my cloud drive. This photo-of-a-photo stands for what I have lost this year—the ability to seek companionship at times of loss.

Rafadi Hakim

LISTEN TO NATURE! (FIG. 3.8)

While humans have been told to stay away from each other, to keep a distance, to wear a mask, and to stay home as much as possible since March 2020, many have not been following this advice. It is understandable, since we are sociable beings and need to be in touch with each other. Isolation and solitude are hard to bear. As Albert Camus wrote in *La Peste* ("The Plague"), "*dans ces extrémités de la solitude, enfin, personne ne pouvait espérer l'aide du voisin et chacun restait seul avec sa préoccupation*" ("in these extremities of solitude nobody could count on any help from their neighbor; each had to bear the load of their own preoccupations alone").[2] We need to be able to be in isolation to survive COVID-19. Nature has spoken clearly lately in the Southern Tier, for example. This area of New York State usually sees snowstorms with a snow accumulation of 12–20 inches. However, on December 17, 2020, the Southern Tier was hit hard by a snowstorm: there was an unexpected accumulation of 42 inches of snow, and all of it in one night. People found themselves stuck in their homes, with no way to get out. Even their mailboxes were stuck and iced under four feet of snow. No temptations to go to restaurants, to meet with friends, to party for the holidays. As soon as a small path was created in the snow, after hours and hours of shoveling and plowing, moreover, the large street plowers were blocking houses and covering mailboxes again. Just stay home!

Sabina M. Perrino

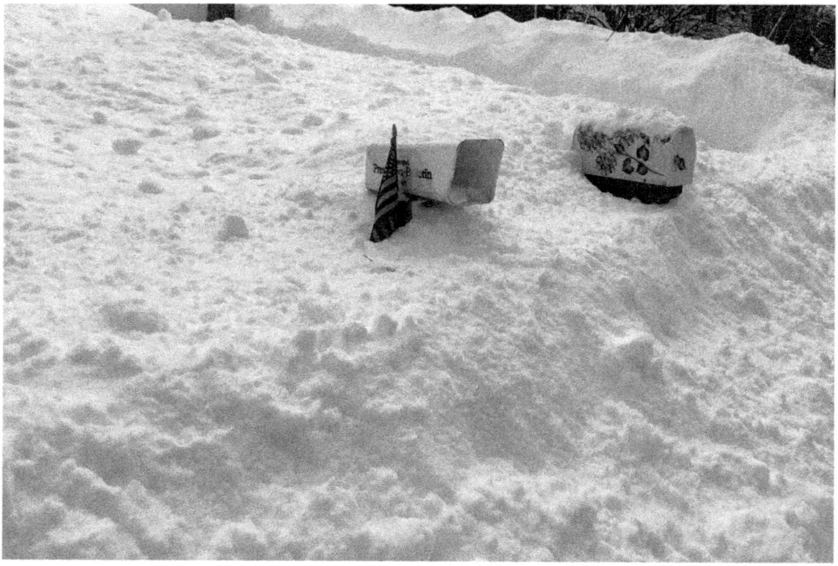

Fig. 3.8 After a snowstorm, Vestal, New York. December 18, 2020. (Photo by S. M. Perrino)

Getting Ready for a Lonely New Year's Eve Party (Fig. 3.9)

December 31, 2020. In a deserted department store, a customer is having her makeup done by beautician clad in anti-contagion protective gear.

Aurora Donzelli

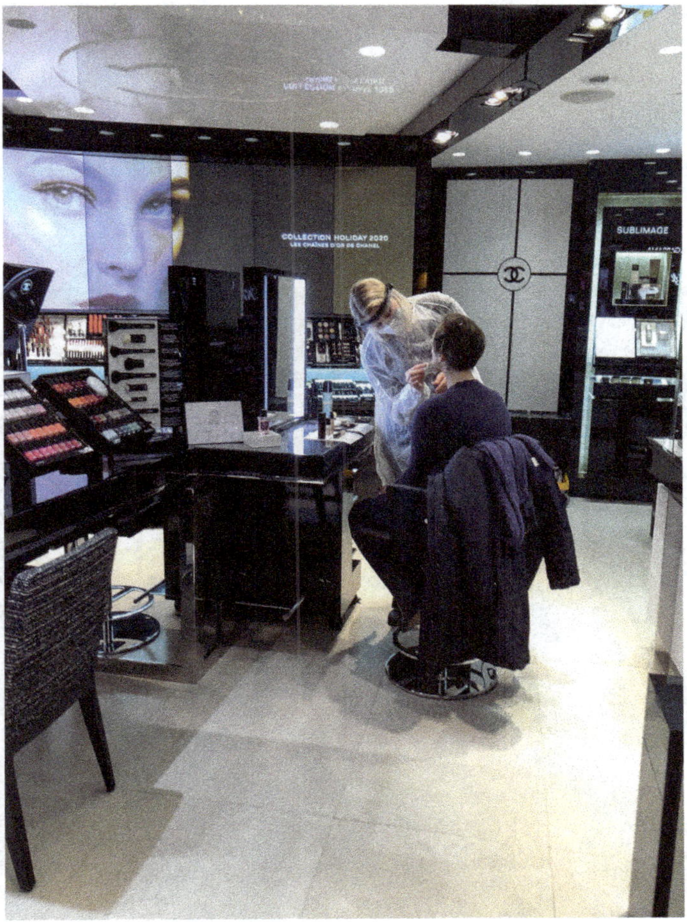

Fig. 3.9 Department store La Rinascente, Milan, Italy. (Photo by A. Donzelli)

Creation Destruction Creation... (Fig. 3.10)

There are mobile testing sites popping up everywhere around us, mostly in unused but central locations. This one, situated behind the sign, is temporarily located in a local park in Binghamton that we used to frequent with our son, called Our Space. This part of Rec Park became known for its up-to-date, disability-friendly equipment, which gave us a sense of pride in our community, and which our son (who has an autism diagnosis) enjoyed when he felt like going out. It is also, incidentally, the site of a carousel that featured as a central plot device in Rod Serling's *Twilight Zone* episode, *Walking Distance* (originally aired October 30, 1959) that allows a disillusioned man to go back in time to the community he grew up in and see himself as a contented child. Serling, that plaque informs, grew up in Binghamton.

Then came the fire. It happened just after Black Lives Matter protesters peacefully marched past the park and downtown to the government and

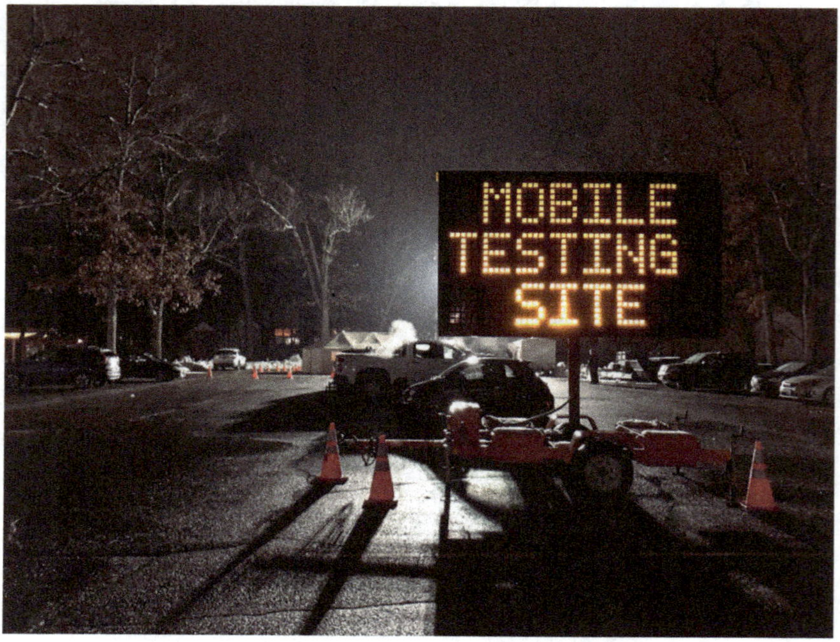

Fig. 3.10 Mobile Testing Site. (Photo by J. Reno)

legal buildings, the biggest such protest, locally, after the murder of George Floyd sparked outrage across the country. Much later that night, the first of June, three days before our son's birthday, someone set fire to the disability-friendly playground equipment and it burned away like kindling. I didn't know that playgrounds could burn like that. If I'm honest, I was more upset at the prospect that opponents of racial justice and police reform would use the fire as an excuse to label the peaceful protests as "violent riots." Local media has been careful to distance the fire from the protests that happened, thankfully. It is still unknown who started the fire, or why. I know this much: they decided to burn something new, something built in 2016, rather than something old, the Rod Serling merry-go-round. I think that choice is less out of respect for the old Binghamton and more about where money and values lie today, in the new Binghamton. Or maybe they just thought the playground would burn easier. As Gaston Gordillo writes, in *Rubble: the Afterlife of Destruction*, "the difference between spatial destruction and production is, to a large degree, in the eyes of the beholder."[3]

The husk of the old playground remained there, a charred and broken ruin, for months as citizens and businesses hurriedly raised money for the rebuild, which began in August and was finished in October. It is good as new, or so I've read. We haven't been back, not since COVID numbers started to go up again and the prospect of going out seemed less appealing. The closest I've been to the playground since just after the fire was when I took this picture, on the 4th of January. In the meantime, the newly constructed site has become one of the county's selected settings for a temporary, emergency mobile testing site.

When they first were building Our Space, four years ago, the sponsors of the playground had to have volunteers stand guard around the equipment to prevent vandalism. Attacks on the playground equipment didn't start with the fire in 2020, in other words. It has occurred to me that the mobile site, open all hours, this week only, might temporarily prevent another fire, but who can know for sure.

Out of destruction, creation.

Josh Reno

Tree Disposal (Fig. 3.11)

The Christmas tree needs to go—it is dried out and shedding everywhere. Curbside collection isn't happening this year. I set out with my children for a designated pickup spot at a nearby park with the tree taking a child's spot in the stroller. The exact location turns out to be at 123rd, a longish walk in the rain. The kids are complaining but I don't want to dump it on the side of the street. As we continue our increasingly grim walk, my

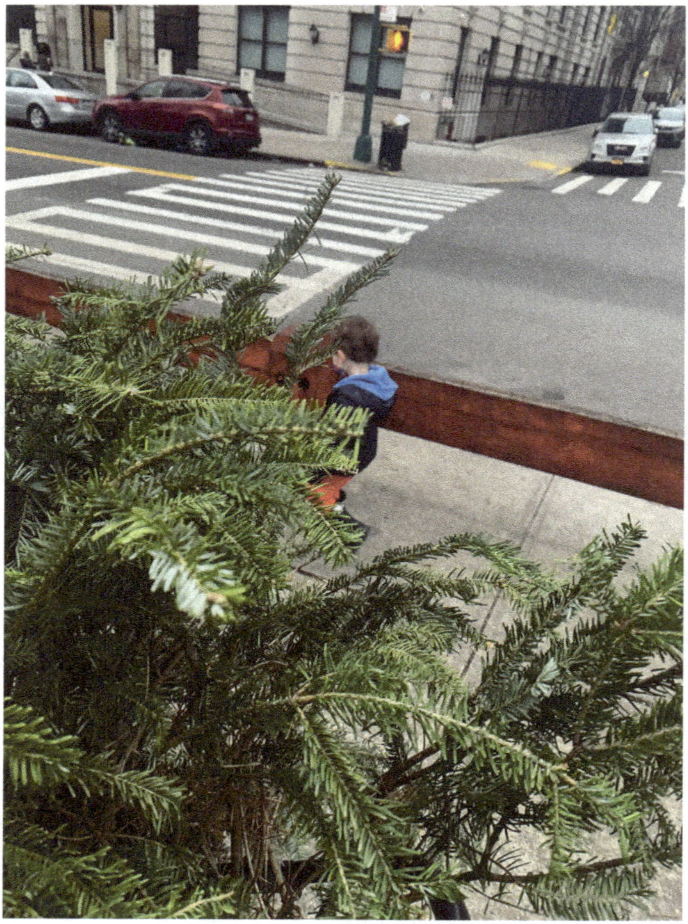

Fig. 3.11 The Goodbye March. (Photo by N. Bartlett)

three-year-old son, for several months an incorrigible mask refuser, wears his without complaining, a small victory of the last months of 2020. We arrive at the drop-off spot, and add ours to perhaps 100 other trees that sit in a pile along the fence. We are cold and wet, and the kids are grumpy, but our tree has been disposed of properly. It will be mulched and find its way into the parks instead of sitting indefinitely amidst holiday trash in some landfill. In this moment, this seems an important way to start the year.

Nicholas Bartlett

Winter Evening in Savoy, Illinois (Fig. 3.12)

Marking the passage of time during COVID is very confusing. The days and weeks and even months blur together, and it still feels like March 2020 never ended. The days carry no distinct memories as far as work is concerned. Routines are identical from day to day, and it feels as though our bodies are stuck in time, fossilized in amber waiting to be freed and brought back to life again. The seasons changed but without the usual fanfare of outdoor activities and gatherings, we only see them through the glass windows of home and the car. Decorations outside of neighbor's homes—for Halloween and Christmas—remind us of holidays that came and went, yet through it all I can't help but feel like we have hardly moved or changed.

Except for our daughter. She's just turned fourteen months, and continues to change faster than we can keep up. My body aches at the end of each day, from trying to play with her, carrying her, and keeping her occupied. She has become the only real signal for the passage of time, but a profound one. Often in the simplest and most mundane of things—such as her reaching out to touch the window of the car as we pull up to a stop sign, where just weeks before she could hardly touch the car door, or her sudden ability to climb down from our bed without any help—we find reminders that it has indeed been more than a year since she's been in our lives.

Parthiban Muniandy

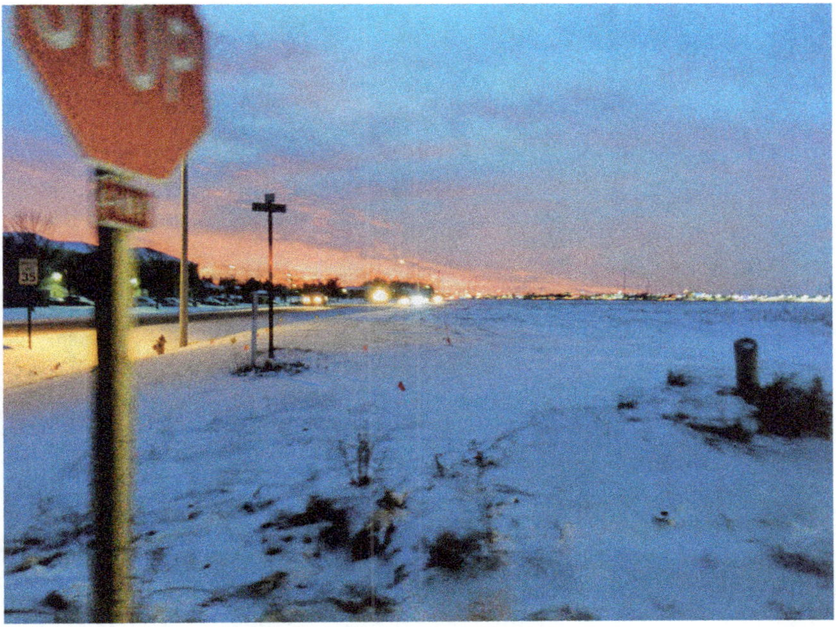

Fig. 3.12 Winter Evening in Savoy, Illinois. January 1, 2021. (Photo by P. Muniandy)

Notes

1. Benjamin (2016: 89–90).
2. Camus (1947: 74).
3. Gordillo (2014: 114).

CHAPTER 4

Part IV: Calculations

We are now asking ourselves to write about our daily "calculations" in COVID-19 times. Spatiotemporal dimensions have been altered by the pandemic, and so are our ways to calculate our daily activities. Whether we calculate the moments of our days and how slow or fast they are, the spaces that separate us from our loved ones or from those who have died, the distance of our encounters with other humans as a reassurance to have avoided a possible contagion, calculations have been a key part of our (un)conscious everyday life. Do we pay more attention to calculations because we are now part of a society struggling through a pandemic of unprecedented proportions? In what ways do we calculate our actions, thoughts, deeds, emotional stances on a daily basis? Are calculations a way to soothe our worried souls?
January 2021

Viral Load

"You're infected with the coronavirus. But how infected?" So goes the title of a recent *New York Times* article, which reports that doctors working in hospitals in the United States are now being encouraged to take into account the estimated "viral load" of patients that come into their care as a way to determine the status of the sick, and to assess which patients "are more likely to deteriorate quickly, and which are most likely

R. Desjarlais et al., *Dispatches from Home and the Field during the COVID-19 Pandemic*, Palgrave Studies in Literary Anthropology, https://doi.org/10.1007/978-3-031-19193-0_4

to fight off the virus and to recover."[1] The scientific research is relatively new on such emergent knowledge, and much is still unclear, but it appears that such estimates and "Ct counts" will come to weigh into the many, ever-shifting calculations that health care workers draw on in treating patients afflicted with the virus.

Calculations of my own come into play with each new day of the pandemic, with decisions that need to be made and questions to be answered, minor, pressing, or with potentially long-term consequences. To cite just a few:

(a) Should I drive up to Massachusetts for Thanksgiving—and then again for Christmas—to spend a few days with my eighty-five-year-old mother and family there, or should I heed the cautionary warnings of Dr. Antony Fauci and other public health experts, and the pleas of exhausted nurses and doctors, to not travel during the holidays, nor join in on any collective celebrations this time round, to keep the viral counts low?
(b) Should I hold my courses completely online when I return to teaching this spring, or should I adopt a hybrid model, with some actual physical presence on campus?
(c) How often should I purchase and wear new masks? Relatedly, how often should I keep recycling and re-using the masks already in my possession?
(d) How often should I go in person to stores to shop for food and other essentials? How often should I order online, for deliveries to my home?
(e) What time of day should I go to Trader Joe's, or Whole Foods, to pick up food for the week? How careful do I need to be while there? How close should I stand to others while waiting in the check-out at Whole Foods?
(f) When can I expect to receive one of the new vaccinations, based on my age, profession, health status, and any chronic health concerns?
(g) Should I consider going to any restaurants (seated inside, or outside?), bars, music venues, film theaters, bookstores? Should I consider making a trip to New York City (by train or automobile?)—to meet up with friends that I have not seen for a while? Would I feel comfortable taking the subway while in the city?
(h) Should I return to the gym and begin to work out again? If so, what days, times, and activities would be safest for that? What kind of exercise can I safely undertake these days?

(i) What are my chances of contacting the virus, and getting sick, if I _______ [fill in the blank with any number of possible activities]?
(j) If I do fall ill with the virus, what are the odds that the illness will be a serious and lasting one? What are the chances that I would lose my sense of smell and taste (as some have)? What are the odds that I, you know, might ____ (die)?
(k) How different or similar am I—in terms of age, sex, profession, health status, lifestyle, viral load intake—from the person who died yesterday, as reported on the news?
(l) Should I go to the trouble of preparing a new last will and testament?
(m) How often should I go out, to be around other people? How long can I last on my own in the reclusive shelter of my apartment, in isolation, without the actual, physical presence of others? How long can I be on my own, away from others, before everything starts to dissolve into a plenum of despondent nothingness?

These and other questions tumble through my mind most days. Each prospect requires a calculation of its own, a tentative guesswork estimation of the risks, possibilities, numbers, statistics, and pinball ricochet chances involved with each encounter, situation, space, moment, or plan. One calculates, counts, measures the risks, without knowing at all what's really involved. It's like a multitude of algorithms are silently, mysteriously at work, but no one can truly access the codes or principles of these algorithms with any clarity or insight.

One constant scene of calculation, for me and others, is the café I like to go to in Dobbs Ferry, one of the river towns set along the eastern banks of the Hudson River, north of New York City. Caffe Latte is owned and managed by an amiable, witty man from Rome named Basilio; he's the only one who works there, twelve hours a day six days a week. Many locals and a few recurrent visitors have made the café a frequent destination in their lives; along with the excellent coffees and foods, many, like myself, find it a place of warmth and friendly conviviality, and we return again and again to this "fine establishment" for fine espressos, cappuccinos, casual conversations, and lasting friendships.

All this has been threatened by the pandemic. For one, the seating is now limited, per the public health orders of the New York State Board of Health. Several of the tables are marked with signs noting that they cannot be used. Six feet apart is the rule, which Basilio abides. People are anxiously aware of what being inside a relatively small place, among others, might entail (Fig. 4.1).

When I returned to the States in early November 2020, after being in Europe the previous eight months, I started to go to the café again. I craved the warm and inviting atmosphere there; better than being always alone at home, I reasoned. But I knew with each breath that there were risks involved. I soon found I had to calculate how often I should go there; where I should sit when there; whether or not I should wear a mask while seated and sipping on a savored macchiato; and how long I should stay for, with each visit. I've found myself going there most afternoons, for an hour or two—for better or worse. It's an uneven trade-off, and delicate balancing act: companionship, at the risk of getting sick or infecting others. The welcome presence of people; the feared circulation of the virus. If possible, I try to sit at table to the side, near one of the windows, potentially a good space away from others—the magical "six feet distance" alive

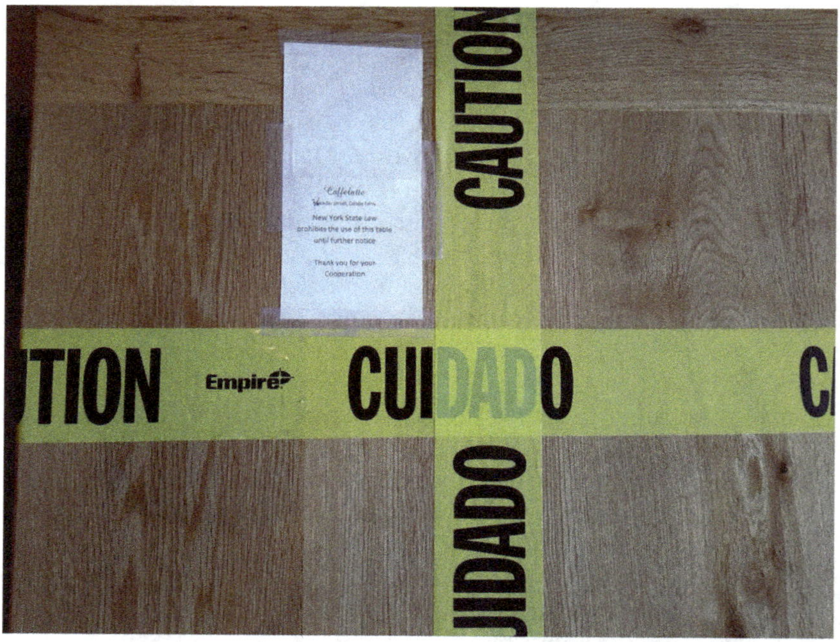
CAUTION
Caffelatte
New York State Law
prohibites the use of this table
until further notice
Thank you for your
Cooperation
TION
Empire
CUIDADO
CUIDADO

Fig. 4.1 Notice affixed to a table at a café in Dobbs Ferry, New York. February 2021. (Photo by R. Desjarlais)

in my mind. But still. Particles are in the air. There is a risk I know in going there most days, though I'm not sure what the algorithms for this are. Anxiety quickly sets in if someone steps close to me, especially if that person is not wearing a mask. The open mouth of a chatty visitant looms monstrous at times.

I can tell others are also anxious. Most are calculating the risks involved, here and there, and possibly there—but not there, no way—as they progress through their days. Most people try to keep their distance from other mortals while at the cafe. Others have stopped coming to the cafe altogether. Some dart in and out. A few appear oblivious to any viral concerns at all. Many enter the place but only to order coffees "to go." Basilio tries to serve them quickly, to cut down on the numbers of people inside, standing close to each other. A few regulars will enjoy their coffees while seated or standing outside the café; they try to keep any time spent inside to a minimum. One wintry afternoon, though not especially cold, I caught the eye of one man as he was walking out the door with two coffees in his hands, the second for his wife, who was standing outside, bundled in a winter coat. We nodded as he passed. At the open door he turned and said to me, "I'd like to sit inside—but I have twenty years on you." Meaning that, as he was twenty years older than me, he had to be more cautious about the risks involved.

One can nearly see the numbers being calculated.

"I want to get Covid," I heard a woman say one day. She was seated at a nearby table, with her young daughter. "I want to get the virus. I'm tired of worrying about it all the time."

This is the other kind of viral load that many of us carry these days.

The other day I read that one-out-of-every-seventy persons in the United States has been infected with the virus. If that's the case, and if I encounter some ten to twenty or thirty people at the café each time I'm there, then what are the chances that one or two of them are infected with the virus, at any given moment? Do the math.

We are moths drawn to a flame.

"It's all about reducing risk," said one café regular in reflecting on the calculus one day. Reducing risk can also mean reductions in life more generally.

One Saturday afternoon I mentioned such concerns to Cate, another frequent café-goer. Cate, who lives with her family in Dobbs Ferry, used to stop by the café once or twice each day to have a leisurely coffee while reading the paper, and to chat with Basilio and say hello to other regulars. This was in pre-pandemic times. Since the contagions of COVID-19 struck New York State with devastating force this year she has cut down on her visits. She always wears a mask while there, even while seated by herself. She'll take it off only momentarily, when taking a sip from the cappuccino set before her. (She is more careful than I am, in that respect.) I've noticed that Cate always wears a KN95 respirator mask, which is to say of the kind of woven fabric that serves to protect herself from the virus, not just others. On that Saturday I stepped into the café and saw that Cate was seated by herself at a table toward the rear of the café. I waved hello to her—from a distance. And then, walking closer to where she was seated, standing some five or six feet away—aware of the near encroachment on the tentative security of her chosen space—I said hello. I told her that I might be writing a brief essay on "calculating during the pandemic," and situating my reflections within the context of the café. "Oh good," she said. "It's about time someone wrote about this place." We were both wearing masks; for the first time I noticed the color of her eyes. I explained what I had in mind—the many calculations we make in our everyday lives—and suggested that perhaps she could give some thought to the matter, and then get back to me at some point, possibly when we next saw each other at the café. "Okay, that sounds good," she said.

Twenty minutes later, while I was seated at a table near the front windows, Cate walked close to me. "I've just jotted some things down, on my phone," she said. "Let me send them to you by text." She did just that, and then left the café. I read her words soon after. This is what she wrote:

> *Covid Calculations*
> Which of my friends are "trustworthy" to spend time with without worrying?
> What constitutes a bubble? If it is malleable, is it safe, or must it remain rigid? Inconsistencies in attitudes of people in bubble (flip-flopping between hyper risk-adverse and flexibility).
> Protecting the mental health of college-age daughter studying remotely from home—her need for socialization vs our need to maintain physical health.
> We're pretty risk-averse. But seeing our daughter who lives in L.A. requires her to take a plane. We make an exception for that risk (twice).
> Agreeing to have 94-year-old mother-in-law have her favorite aide come every day, even though the aide also works in a nursing home that has had

Covid cases (the aide quarantines if she is ever exposed). Safety of visiting mother-in-law even though aide comes every day.

Never going to a restaurant or friend's house or anywhere inside, but going to the café every day because it's such an important part of my life. Calculation is to sit separately from others, wear my mask the whole time and never stay longer than ½ hour. It's a false sense of security to put these rules into place for myself, but it allows me to do the thing I want to do with impunity.

With such calculations, ongoing, ever-changing, recombinant, other factors are now being thrown into the mix. How will the emergence of any new, more contagious strands of the virus—or, alternatively, the introduction of nationwide vaccination campaigns—alter the silent algorithms at work?

Robert Desjarlais

COVID-19 Daily Spatiotemporal Calculations

December 20, 2020

My phone is ringing. I usually don't let my phone ring for unknown callers. They are silenced. Only my phone contacts have the privilege to make my phone ring. I decided to set up my phone in this way a couple of years ago when my phone number was hacked and I had to change it as a result. I smile when I see Sophia's name appearing on my phone screen.

"Hi Sophia, how are you?"

"Hi Sabina! Are you there? Are you home?"

"No, I'm not home right now, but I'm walking home. I took a short walk in the snow and will be home in 10 minutes."

"That's perfect. I am driving to Vestal. I would like to stop by. I have to drop off something."

"Do you have something for me? You didn't need to do that!" I said while smiling behind my light-blue face mask.

"No, no, no, don't worry!" said Sophia. "I just have a little something for you. I will be there in 10 minutes."

I can't believe it. Sophia is coming to my place. The last time she came to see me was in April 2020, soon after the lockdown in New York State.

At that time, she had just started to offer fitness Zoom classes to all her gym members and she wanted to give me some extra sliding discs for some exercises. She also wanted to see where I live. "Just in case," she said, "just in case we need to help each other." She was afraid. While I walk back home fast, I try to vividly experience those past moments again through mental spatiotemporal shifts. Those moments are so far away in time and space. All these past months still seem so unreal. And, yet, she decided to visit me today. Of course, as it happened back in April, we won't be able to sit down on my couch, inside my apartment. We can only see each other in the parking lot, very quickly, by precisely calculating the distance between us and by wearing our face masks. We have been both very cautious, very respectful, we haven't broken the rules. We have made our own, careful, daily calculations. I was supposed to pick up something from her backyard porch last week, and I went there when she was not home. I knew she was not there. I planned it. COVID-19 has forced us to follow some schemes and routes we couldn't even imagine a year ago. We have been avoiding each other with mastery.

I need to hurry up. I'm looking at the time on my phone. She said she would be "there" in 10 minutes. I have to walk fast. 10 minutes might not be enough time for me. I need to speed up. I am happily anxious. I'll see her in a three-dimensional way; I haven't seen her in so long. Yet, I see her through my computer screen almost every day. I safely take her fitness classes from home now. I exercise mask-free from the comfort of my living room. It has been fun and meaningful. She now has developed a real business, which started from nothing. I make my calculations through time and space, I go back with my memory to remember how she was in person, her eyes with fake eye-lashes, her way of walking, her way of interacting, her demeanor. I walk even faster now. I don't want to be late at our improvised rendezvous. It's five minutes away. I should be able to make it. I won't be able to go inside my apartment to warm a bit my hands. I'm freezing. It's really cold today. Twenty degrees Fahrenheit with a strong wind. There is so much snow around me. It is just difficult to walk fast on and in the snow. We had a big snowstorm three days ago. There are walls of snow all around me.

I feel happiness in my heart. I will see Sophia after so long. Perhaps she felt bad that she was not home when I went to her backyard porch the other day. She doesn't know that it was a calculation of mine to avoid the temptation to chat for hours inside her home. It is too cold outside to be on a porch anyway. Temptation would have been a winner. Temptation doesn't follow our calculated decisions or manners. It was better to follow my calculations. A very difficult and very different Christmas this year. That's the holiday I usually celebrate with my family elsewhere. I see Sophia's car approaching. I made it to the parking lot at the perfect, calculated time. I just wave from afar. I see her hand waving back inside her car. A few feet are separating us now. She has no mask on and she lowers her car window. I can see her face, she smiles and seems happy. I smile back, but she cannot see my full smile. She can read my excitement through my eyes, however. A new way to read non-verbal communication in COVID-19 times: through the different ways we stretch our eyes. I wear my mask all the time when I'm out. It's too dangerous not to. There are too many people who are not wearing it around where I live. They don't seem to care. For them, the virus is a hoax; it doesn't exist. In their perspective, it is a (mis)calculation to disrupt our life. That is what the manager of my rental complex thinks. Sophia and I look at each other straight in the eyes. The eyes communicate much more than words. Emotions can be enacted and seen through eyes. She says a few words from the window of her car. With a calculated effort, and avoiding the direct exposure to me, she hands me a small package which looks like a Christmas gift. It is elegantly wrapped in green paper with a golden ribbon on it. This is the second Christmas gift I've received this year. I hope she can't see my eyes getting full of tears. That is pure, uncalculated happiness.

Sabina M. Perrino

The Calculi of Pleasure

"This is a great time to invest in eyes." Flabbergasted, I look at the stranger standing in front of me. I scramble to make sense of her odd blunt statement. On my way back from a trip to the municipal headquarters to settle some unpaid trash collection fees, I walked by La Rinascente—an historic department store in downtown Milan. I had no design to make a shopping detour while running my end-of-the-year errands, but the sight of some commercial activity in a non-essential store caught my attention.

Incredulous, I walk closer and discover that La Rinascente is actually open for business, in spite of the New Year's Eve lockdown measures. I express my surprise to the muscular security guard standing in front of the store entrance and I am courteously told that only the beauty stores located on the ground floor are exempt from the red zone measures enforced by the Italian government during the holidays. "They are considered akin to pharmacies," adds the guard in response to my bewildered gaze.

Having spent almost two hours discussing with a municipal clerk the unpleasant matter pertaining to unpaid trash fees and fines I unwittingly inherited from a distant relative who died years ago, I find myself inexorably driven to the phantasmagoric world of cosmetics and makeup. I push my way through the two sets of heavy glass doors in search of some distraction from the anxiety generated by my newly discovered trash debts. After plunging into the bureaucratic meanders of municipal revenue services, I re-emerge into the dreamy landscape of a ghost-town shopping mall. A soft-white glow embraces me as I begin to wander through the corridors created by the artful arrangement of makeup kiosks and cosmetic display counters. I am immediately reminded of the pleasure given by the soothing, near-hypnotic effect of the warmed-toned lighting designed to minimize skin imperfections. I cannot recall the last time I entertained myself with the beauty store flânerie that used to constitute an occasional pastime of mine before the pandemic. Although the lights and layout have remained unchanged, a new store policy forbids customers from touching and testing the products. As I dawdle in a dream-state, I only gradually realize that I am the only human presence, aside from one other customer and the salespersons standing by each brand counter. Feeling observed, I suddenly awake from my trance-like purposeless wandering: "How much is it?" I ask, trying to look like a normal customer, although I have no real interest in buying the fancy eyeliner my finger is pointing at. "Forty-one Euros." I remain unresponsive. The sales representative—perhaps interpreting my pensive reaction to the price she has given me as a symptom of a customer's indecisiveness— repeats her odd blunt statement: "This is a great time to invest in eyes." As try to I re-emerge from my somnambulatory limbo, I look at her masked face and her meticulously made-up false-lashed eyes and finally understand the subtle irony underlying her commercial pun. "That's all we have left," she adds in a more somber tone.

I often think of my many lost little pleasures, wondering if they are lost forever. Indulging in aimless window shopping, wasting time trying on new makeup in a department store, eating an ice-cream cone while chatting with a friend, going for a swim at the pool and hanging out in the steam room afterwards, going out for drinks at one of my favorite cocktail bars during a crowded Milanese happy hour, eating out, cooking dinner for friends, or, simply walking savoring the day without having to wear a facemask.

> The more the virus replicates itself by infecting more humans the greater the chance the virus will mutate and develop more competitive variants, which will drastically reduce the vaccine efficacy. The virus needs human flesh to replicate itself. We need to get vaccinated en mass as soon as possible to deprive this virus of its humus.[2]

The words of a famous immunologist come out of my radio a few days before Christmas, while Europe is under the new wave of panic caused by the discovery of the more infective UK strain. In front of the magnitude of such horrendous threats, I have become unable to pursue my modest ordinary pleasures. I feel entrapped in a clash of scales: on the one hand, the big statistical numbers of relative risk calculations; on the other hand, the apparently negligible uniqueness of my small ephemeral pleasures. Numerical computation has infested the domain of moral reasoning and practical judgment: statistical analysis and algorithmic calculations now dominate our daily speculations about how to live wisely and well.

I miss the ordinary amusements of my old life, but I seem unable to embrace a statistical approach to the new COVID-related dialectic of risk and pleasure and carve for myself an adaptive niche. Take the example of the maximum of six people per table—a safety measure that has traveled from the realm of commercial dining to that of family gatherings during Thanksgiving and Christmas celebrations. The measures adopted by the government are a perfect illustration of the statistical approach: Why six and not eight or four guests? It takes one person with a high viral load—a super spreader—to infect an entire party of people. Although grounded in a sound statistical calculation, this dining policy has no capacity to ensure individual safety. The statistical approach is an effective tool to ensure relative collective security, but has little meaning if seen from the absolute standpoint of the embodied life (and death) of the individual. And yet the perimeters of risk assessment have gradually infected my daily reasoning, which is now unfolding in a new economy of moral and causal scales. I often catch myself entertaining somewhat pitiable thoughts. What shall I do if a friend asks me what in a COVID-free world would be an ordinary and easily granted favor, such as staying at my place for a couple of nights or getting help packing up for a move? Or, even more prosaically, how can I politely refuse an invitation to have dinner at the home of an old friend, who has three exuberant kids? Although I recognize the pettiness of my thoughts, I am unable to dismiss them.

The new modes of risk assessment reasoning have restructured human sociality. There is an emotional disjuncture of sorts in individuals' perceptions of risk. More than the injunction to social distance, the pandemic-induced calculative reasoning has fractured human relations, creating deep but invisible disconnections between new social types. Once upon a time there were the introverts and the extroverts and in spite of occasional misunderstandings they could complement each other, finding meaningful forms of intimacy. Now new polarizations have emerged between the risk-adverse and the risk-defiant, the careful and the reckless, the compliant and the disobedient, the conspiracy-minded anti-vaxxers and the pro-science advocates. Unlike the many possible intersections that were once possible between perceptive and insightful loners and carefree gregarious extroverts, now there seems to be little room for interaction between the new human types that have emerged in response to the give and take of pandemic everyday life.

Some people seem more comfortable with statistical exercises, while others (like myself) are more inclined to an all-or-nothing approach to pleasure, friendship, and love. But how long can this last? How long can old-time friendships tolerate the disappointments created by different sensitivities to COVID-related matters? How long can intimacy survive at a distance? How long can non-cohabiting lovers stay apart before becoming totally estranged from each other? How long can phone and video calls replace physical contact?

The words of another prominent epidemiologist interviewed on the radio provide a gloomy scenario: in light of the currently projected average of 60,000 people inoculated per day, we need to consider that we have 60 million Italians to vaccinate, which divided by 60,000 vaccinations a day makes about 1000 days. However, since Pfizer and AstraZeneca require two doses for the vaccine to be effective, we have to calculate 1000 days x 2, that is, 2000 days, which means that it will take 4–5 years before Italy's entire population gets vaccinated.[3]

Aurora Donzelli

2021

Numbers often have a hard time holding my attention when they multiply. Although their particular shapes and combinations do at times strike me in their implication or beauty, and although I too have tried to deploy the charisma of numbers now and then in writing or in banter, the exhibition of numbers, including their proliferation since the arrival of the once-unnamed virus, often leaves me with a peculiar empty feeling. This is not to claim precedence of the sentimental over the calculable, or even to contrast measure with meaning. Nor is it quite to say (or quite to oppose) what psychologist Paul Slovic said of Americans' numbness toward COVID-19 death tolls: "Statistics are human beings with tears dried off;" "In fact, the more who die, sometimes the less we care."[4] It is maybe to sit with the way that numbers start to lose their initial force on me, while producing a different kind of force, in their escalation, repetition, and emptying out. A funeral casino, as Alan Klima put it, writing of mass death in Thailand.[5] I, like "countless" others perhaps, find myself softly hypnotized by the slippage and blurring of attention amid growing numbers, as well as their punctuation by the ones that stick. A quick search for "death toll" in headlines since the beginning of this new year brings, for instance:

> *"Illinois' pandemic death toll surpasses 17,500."*
> *"California's coronavirus death toll approaches 30K."*
> *"New Mexico's COVID-19 death toll increases by 17."*
> *"UK coronavirus cases top 3 million as death toll passes 80,000."*
> *"As coronavirus death toll surpasses 350,000, Trump calls U.S. count 'far exaggerated.'"*[6]

And then, since March of last year:

> *"Six feet."*

There is a strangeness in the pairing. It is, of course, not so simple. The counting of death is triangulated with many other numbers: ICU capacities, viral loads, thresholds for herd immunity, numbers allowed to gather beyond the household unit, numbers allowed to gather in public, days of quarantine, pending vaccine availability, measured in months, years, doses. All these numbers continue to shift; all these numbers have their formulae. Many work hard to refine them; many plot their coordinates of duty and care around them. Meanwhile, I, like many others around me, take my not-so-precisely-calculated risks, complemented by their attendant gestures. I stroll through my neighborhood, vaguely wondering whether to shift that extra foot or two away at the sight of oncoming walkers, while mirroring their minor facial signals and contortions—that small avoidance of the gaze which lives at the border of courtesy and embarrassment, that diplomatic acknowledgment of a small nod, that look of anxiety bordering on disgust. The one-or-two-foot elliptical swoop paired with the face of the moment—stylized elaborations on a probabilistic recommendation. Six feet—is it this? I do this and many other things big and small, in which the logic of numbers begin to slip and fall, and living is no longer secured by the numbers, even if the numbers may have first offered some scaffolding. Instead, the days come to be hosted by gestures and excesses parasitic of such numeric infrastructure, or at times falling out of them entirely.

I write this four days after Trump supporters "stormed the Capitol"—their own phrasing which is said to have been used 100,000 times online the month before the event. Here is a headline, for good measure:

> *"Death toll from mob's storming of US Capitol rises to 4, DC police say."*[7]

I write this five days after someone in my extended family died with the virus after living with it for over 40 days. A death toll of 1, a number with its own peculiar force, which brings on an emptying out in its own peculiar style.

I don't quite know what to make of these new numbers yet. Nor the ones that came before. It's 2021.

Emily Ng

Vaccine on the Mind

On Monday morning, I receive a text from a colleague at the university. Over the weekend, the city announced new plans to ease a bottleneck in early attempts to vaccinate medical workers. We had entered "Phase 1b." I follow the link in my friend's message, check a box noting that I am an "education worker," and fill out a few other questions. In less than five minutes, I have an appointment in 10 days at a facility less than a mile from my office.

The vaccine has suddenly transformed from a distant harbinger of a post-pandemic era to a concrete appointment in my calendar. With my spot in line so quickly assured, I become uneasy. Why should I be in this round? Was it a mistake? Maybe I should cancel and allow someone else at greater risk of infection to take my spot. On the internet, I find an editorial about a division among House "squad" members Alexandria Ocasio-Cortez and Ilhan Omar, the former an early vaccinator and the later refusing to cut in front of frontline workers. The author observes the spat is part of a new "ugly world" of vaccine distribution that renews attentions to unequal distribution of resources.

Last night, I had a dream. I am coasting on my bicycle down a familiar street. The road I am riding on has changed; what was once a flat stretch is now a hill. At first, I am enjoying an easy, effortless ride. But then, the lights go out. In the dark, there are shadowy bodies in the street. I am not sure if they are alive or dead. The bike's momentum now feels reckless—I've lost control of the breaks. A collision seems inevitable.

Nicholas Bartlett

The Second (And Third) Shift

Four hours. My wife and I use four-hour blocks each day between us to juggle work, childcare, house chores, and leisure. Notwithstanding the weekends, when we do not get the benefit of the daycare, these four-hour blocks are meant to help us buy time for one another to get through teaching, emails, writing and perhaps a shower (a luxury!). For each of those blocks, one of us will be with our daughter while the other gets through, well, everything else. We discuss, plan, and even argue over these four-hour blocks, constantly trying to juggle our shifts along with the other items on our schedule for the day, including meetings, phone calls to family, and other errands. It always starts the same way—who wakes up earlier to take up that first shift in the morning. Usually, it ends up being the person who did not wake up in the middle of the night to help put the baby back to sleep when she wakes up crying for her bottle or because she had a bad dream.

One of the challenges of taking care of a toddler these days is this lack of predictability and sustained routine that allows us to plan, even a day or two ahead. We do not even know who would be the first to wake up, as that often depends on who has the energy to be able to do so after a night of restless and inconsistent sleep. Our plans end up dependent on these four-hour blocks on each day, and during those four hours we often must improvise a sequence of tasks we need to get done. If my shift starts around 11 am on a given day, I'd have to move from feeding the cats, cleaning out their litter, doing the dishes, taking a quick shower, help with the baby's lunch, and use the remaining time to catch up on never-ending emails. If there is any time left after that, I would ideally work on the *actual* labor I spent so much of my adult life looking forward to—working on my teaching material, thinking and writing something *intellectually profound*.

At least that is the ideal sequence of work in theory. Usually, it goes more like this. Upon the start of my four-hour block without the baby, I would try to get the house chores done. Feeding cats and cleaning out the litter would be the easy part. Then comes the attempt to take a shower before realizing, "damn it, there's a full laundry basket in the corner," or "damn it, the kid's room stinks because of the dirty diapers in her waste basket," or "shoot, mom's calling to say hi and see the baby," and before I know it, a couple of hours or more will pass, before I even get to take the shower and feed myself. What time is left, as much as I'd try to dedicate to being "productive," it often ends up being a bit of procrastination playing a video game (I always tell myself I need the break, or I'd risk getting hyper-stressed) followed by an extended blank stare at the computer as I scroll through the endless emails trying to make sense of the words.

Often, at the end of these four-hour blocks, often, I end up feeling like I've done far less than I'd hoped to. That becomes a source of anxiety and frustration that bleeds into impatience and the inability to enjoy the "other" four-hour block of time during the day, which is the time I get to spend fully dedicated to our little girl. Through no fault of hers, she ends up with a parent who is not all there, whose mind keeps going back to that annoying task or thing that he had needed to do but didn't get to, that recommendation letter he had to write but couldn't finish in time, the meeting link he had to create and send out to students but didn't, the email to a colleague he'd needed to write, or a report that was due soon, but he hadn't even started. Through no fault of her own, she ends up with a parent who cannot just put all of that out of his mind and just focus on playing with her, teaching her new things, taking her for a walk, or just spending time *being with her*.

I tell myself that there is no point in feeling these daily frustrations—we can only do what we can, and we are not machines. We can't turn on the productivity switch whenever we want, and we most definitely can't convince our biological and chemical internals to conform to this type of daily scheduling of time. Especially as academics, we tend to be so dependent on what sociologist Annette Lareau[8] called "unplanned time" to be able to do our best forms of thinking, reflecting, and writing. I have gotten used to a way of accomplishing intellectually active labor that involves long blocks of time that are completely devoid of structure and distractions—something that helps me be an ethnographer and writer. It is incredibly difficult to train one's mind and body to condense that notion of time into these semi-routinized but mostly uncertain blocks of time. It becomes near impossible when one is also trying to deal with the attendant anxiety and feelings of parental guilt gnawing constantly at one's innards.

Parenting during COVID, especially as a couple without any immediate family in the same country, has become a constant dance of controlled chaos—always trying to figure out how much time we have during the day to get everything that needs to be done completed, then consistently failing at getting much done, at least in terms of the neoliberal notion of productivity that our careers demand of us. While I recognize the fact that we indeed get through a heck of a lot of work each day, just by taking care of our daughter, feeding her, caring for the emotional well-being of our parents trapped and isolated in our foreign homelands, while trying as much as we can to be supportive partners to one another and keeping our own psyches from going AWOL—it is perhaps a telling symptom of modern life that all that feels hollow and *unproductive* because we end up always measuring ourselves by what we produce rather than what we care for.

Parthiban Muniandy

Calculating a Livelihood

Every time I listen to the radio, I almost always hear numbers that describe how the COVID-19 pandemic has exacerbated global forms of socioeconomic inequality. Although I use the radio as a background for cooking and other household chores, I still notice these numbers, because these numbers resonate with my own experiences. As the pandemic continues to rage, I have experienced a heightened level of financial insecurity—a form of insecurity that demands constant financial calculations and recalculations.

When I listen to public radio hosts who tirelessly explain the economic impact of the pandemic, my mind goes to the calculations I make as I think about my earnings: a combination of a dissertation fellowship and a variety of part-time jobs. Even as elite American universities gradually move toward fully funded models of doctoral education in the past few years, my cohort of graduate students continues to depend on part-time work to make ends meet.

What if there is no teaching assistantship in this writing course next quarter? Should I count on full-time postdoctoral fellowships being available after I submit my dissertation?

I calculated numbers on a spreadsheet that became quite complicated very quickly. This much from an online writing course, this much from a book-writing project, and this much for living expenses.

Should I treat myself with takeout for dinner, one of the few entertainment options available during the pandemic?

The professional academic vision of working on a single book for years at a time seems so far away for me, especially when financial support for dissertation research is often partial, short-term, and relentlessly competitive. I frequently find myself thinking about additional taking jobs unrelated to my dissertation research, because the pandemic seems to have taken a toll on the reliability of universities as a source of income.

Will there be enough students for an additional section that I can teach? Is the number of hours I dedicate to part-time work realistic when I am expected to complete a dissertation?

A public radio program mentioned that high school students who turn eighteen during the pandemic might face unprecedented pressure to start working immediately instead of continuing their education. I started seeing parallels in my own life: after my parents have lost their sources of income early on in the pandemic, financial certainty feels like a much-needed remedy.

I turned my radio off, put my winter coat on, and walked toward Lake Michigan to take a short break from the workday. I thought to myself: thinking about other people, and writing about them, after all, are ways of making a living.

Rafadi Hakim

Notes

1. Apporva Mandavilli. 2020. "You're infected with the Coronavirus. But How Infected?" *New York Times* (https://www.nytimes.com/2020/12/29/health/coronavirus-viral-load.html).
2. Radio interview to Sergio Abrignani, aired on Radiopopolare, during the program *Prisma*, December 21, 2020.
3. Radio interview to Professor Carlo La Vecchia, aired on Radiopopolare, during the program *Prisma*, January 5, 2021.
4. *Washington Post*, "Why Americans are numb to the staggering coronavirus death toll," 12/21/20.
5. Klima (2002).
6. In order (to be formalized at a later point): *Chicago Sun-Times*, *Marin Independent Journal*, *Santa Fe New Mexican*, *Al Jazeera English*, *The Washington Post*.
7. *KPRC 2 News Today*, though the number has grown to 5 at the time of the writing, and now 6 including an officer suicide post-facto; *Mother Jones*, "The phrase 'storm the capitol' was used 100,000 times online in the month leading up to the mob."
8. Lareau (2011).

CHAPTER 5

Part V: Interludes

We are all invited to write an entry by selecting a date in 2021 and thinking back about the same day in 2020. These entries have the function of "Interludes," as ways of reflecting upon how the pandemic has changed human life in exactly one year. How do we see ourselves placed across time and space after a challenging year? What happened on a particular date that we might remember, emotionally, today? What is the significance of revisiting those moments in all their nuances? How different or similar is life after a year into the COVID-19 pandemic?
March 2021

"This Virus Is a Hoax"

March 11, 2021

Today, a year ago, I was getting inundated with dreadful news from my family and friends in Northern Italy where the virus had hit really hard since early February. Some northern Italian regions went into complete lockdown very rapidly. The tolls of contagions and of deaths skyrocketed too. At that time, people didn't really know what to do, how to behave, whether to use face coverings or not, or whether to keep a certain distance from each other. Face masks were not even available for doctors and nurses then. It was, and has been, thoroughly surreal. Since that time, I had been

R. Desjarlais et al., *Dispatches from Home and the Field during the COVID-19 Pandemic*, Palgrave Studies in Literary Anthropology,
https://doi.org/10.1007/978-3-031-19193-0_5

struggling with friends and neighbors in the US, while asking them to follow the required social distancing rules, to wear a mask, and to be careful. When I tried to intervene, everyone would stare at me.

That day, March 11, 2020, as it happens every year, I had a long phone call with my mother, to honor and remember her mother's birthday, my grandma. Every year we tell each other stories and we share memories of her that death cannot remove from us.

"Your grandma would have been over 100 years today," said my Mom with a soothing and sad voice.

"I am at least happy that she didn't need to go through another pandemic," she continued, "she had already survived the Spanish flu, as a little girl, did you know that?"

A year ago, I was not thinking about past pandemics. My grandmother survived the 1918 flu pandemic, World War I and World War II. I was very lucky to have her teachings in my life. Those difficult times are often forgotten.

That day, after my phone call with my mother, I decided to take a walk in the cold breeze of the end of a harsh winter in the Southern Tier, New York. As soon as I stepped out of the main door, I ran into Judy, the manager of my rental complex. As always, she was smoking. I kept my distance from her while I was wearing the only face mask I had. With an antagonist intonation in her voice, she claimed:

"I can't wear those things over my face. I cannot breathe and I don't want to wear them. My Mom gave me a cloth mask, but I won't wear it, period."

Judy seemed to be very upset about the use of masks.

Knowing that in Italy the Government had already asked everyone to wear face masks, I asked her whether she would put informative signs in our rental buildings suggesting to wear a face mask and to keep social distance. Anxiously, and with a grimace on her face, she said:

> "I am not really supposed to make these kinds of suggestions. This is a private property, after all. I won't do it. Plus, do you really believe in this virus? Don't you see what's happening? People have been brainwashed. This virus is a hoax."

Her words petrified me while my glasses were fogging up from the use of my mask. I was speechless, breathing heavily.

I had many meetings with her over this past year. I tried to explain certain facts to her. Judy's beliefs haven't changed. Many tenants in her rental complex share the same ideology. I have never seen them wearing a mask.

Never. They have never seen me without my mask. Never. They don't even know what my face looks like. They will never see my face.

The US has just passed 500,000 COVID-19 related deaths. It is unprecedented. Still, for some people, this virus is a hoax.

Today would have been my grandmother's birthday. I decided to apply two masks since I had to visit Judy in her office. I gave her my last rent check and told her that I will move into my new home by the end of the month.

Sabina M. Perrino

Older Brother

After getting my first Moderna shot, I had to wait for about a half an hour in the community college ice rink to make sure I did not have any strange reactions. I had time to kill, so I called my older brother, who I'd been meaning to reach out to a few days. He and his wife live in North Carolina where, he explained, the state government's refusal to expand Medicare meant they were looking for options to get funding for an MRI for his wife to provide final confirmation of a long-awaited diagnosis of multiple sclerosis. I felt my right arm lightly throb while he expressed the hope that this will bring an end to three decades of uncertainty, pain, prescription drug misuse, and misdiagnosis.

I thought about how we talked about his wife during that hopefully-soon-to-end period of uncertainty, our large and gossipy family, siblings, spouses, children and cousins, and whether we had judged her unfairly because of her medical troubles. Then I thought back to how incensed I got when, a decade before, he'd taken me aside to tell me that their son probably had autism. It felt like the latest ruse, and a cruel one at that. This was just after our son was reintroduced to everyone as now officially severely disabled and we were quite used to how freely his family seemed to self-diagnose for what appeared to be attention, sympathy, and support.

My fists clenched thinking of that moment, one of many reasons that my brother and I had grown apart over the years. I worked hard to push it out of my mind and instead asked him questions about his sons, baby grandchildren, work. I thought about how everyone now thought about health care almost all the time, testing, diagnosis, treatment, cure, quarantine. We were all engaging in forms of "biosociality" in Paul Rabinow's sense, where we are not born with biological imperatives (as in sociobiology) but experience ever new and emergent ways of working on ourselves and being worked on by others in reference to our "nature," including disease.[1] Whether he and his family were seeking attention or answers or both, my brother's life as long as I could remember has been bio-social in this way. This was arguably even more central to their choices and struggles than his fundamentalist Christian ministry, whether his partial deafness and psoriasis, his wife's shifting diagnosis (now lupus, now fibromyalgia, now maybe MS), his eldest son's "PTSD" and his youngest son's schizophrenia (formerly "autism").

"Good luck with the MRI," I said.

Weeks pass and I have had my second shot. I am now fully vaccinated. I call my brother again and it turns out the MRI scan revealed the loss of a myelin sheath and suggests the possibility that his wife is suffering from early onset dementia or Alzheimer's. More tests are needed to rule out MS, which my brother is still hoping for.

If we are all bio-social beings now, my relationship with some friends, relatives, colleagues, and students have always been more obviously marked in that way. Sometimes it seems less strange to talk to my brother than it used to. It's like his world of uncertain and spectacular health is everyone's world now. Sometimes it makes it harder to talk to everyone else. They talk but I hear him, imagine his suspicious motives, feel that peculiar but familiar familial guilt.

Josh Reno

Circling the Year of the Cyclone

March 30, 2021

Exactly a year ago to this day the two of us left our apartment in Crown Heights and rode our bicycles down to the Ferris wheel by the ocean. The slope of Ocean Parkway eased the weariness of the last few weeks of lockdown. Honey locust, London plane, and Norway maple blew in the wind. A siren wailed in the distance. Two black Impalas, engines revving, screamed past us. Fly away hair in her face, Fern yelled, "Assholes!" I cried out in response, "Yeah! But don't you feel a thrill when they blow by?"

I pedaled standing. Under the overpass, onto the sidewalk, eyes squinting, cycling faster until we hit the empty boardwalk. My front tire strikes a stray rock. The rushing sound of the ocean. The spring sun cut to the bone by the chill of a lingering winter wind. We rode slowly weaving through boarded up bumper car rides, shooting galleries, hot dog stands. Circling the cyclone. I laid on my back, photographing the Wonder Wheel, searching the sky, watching the clouds tick past. A heavy fog rolled in off the water. For two hours, it all seemed so unreal. This day was not just another lockdown day, not another domino in a chain of domino days. Just us and Coney Island (Fig. 5.1).

One year later, I was in Tunis for fieldwork. I knocked on the door of a light blue gate. In the street behind me, I heard the voices of two women calling for a taxi, honking, and he groan of a diesel truck. The door swung open and I crossed the threshold into the Jewish cemetery. I walked with Henda, who like her father before her, cares for the twenty thousand dead buried here. The stillness of the space stopped me from asking too many questions. Those would come later, over an orange juice in her sister-in-law's café across the street.

A forest of fig trees had taken root in graves marked with names like Fitoussi, Scemama, Lumbroso, Valensi, and Bellaïche. Their thin branches still winter bare. The earth swallowing stones, bones, and names with

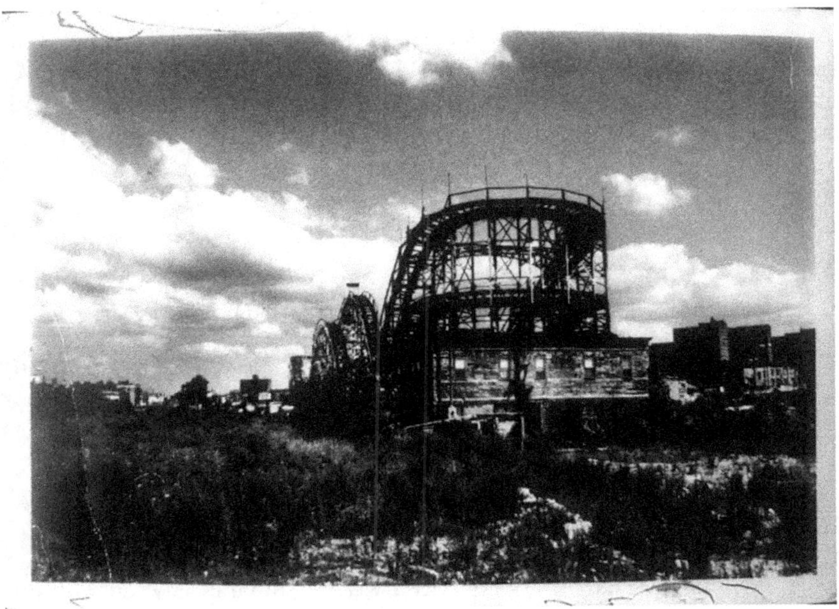

Fig. 5.1 Postcard of Coney Island (1987). The Brooklyn Museum. (Photo by Anita Chernewski © 1990)

barely a whisper. Between the dandelions and blades of grass, a dead butterfly. Its wings fluttered in the wind. We stopped before the BARANES brother's oven-shaped brick tomb. Beside them are Berthe and Léon Fitoussi who, like the baker brothers, died in the early 1950s. Remembering the old Jewish custom of leaving stones at the grave of a loved one, I laid three stones at the foot of their grave. Not my loved ones, but someone's.

Near Henda's small house left of the entrance, her sixteen-year-old nephew and I sat cross-legged on one of the oldest tombs in the cemetery, flat and embedded in the ground as was the custom in Tunisia before French colonization. Only women and children in this section. Epitaphs in Judeo-Arabic and Hebrew. The sun bounced off the white marble. Her nephew and I talked basketball. He pantomimed swishing a jump shot. He didn't miss. The *muezzin* called people to prayer. Cicadas buzzed. I listened to Henda on the phone. Listened to the sparrows. Listened to the cracking in my knees when I stood up to leave.

I walked back to Berthe and Léon Fitoussi's tombstones and slipped the small, opaque, whitish-gray stones into my pocket. To feel the weight of these stones was to feel the presence of Joseph Fitoussi (1931–2020). Each time I slid my hand into my coat, I rubbed their roughness rhythmically, compulsively. Remembrance is a funny thing. It had been one year since my grandfather died of COVID in Paris. And in a year where movement had been limited, where I could not visit his grave in Jerusalem, these pebbles from Tunis, the city where he was born, multiply and fracture. The stones bring me closer to him and to the "shore of dreaming."[2]

Margaux Fitoussi

Memories of March 2020

"Sounds good. I will be done at 9:30. Is Matea going to debut in the faculty dining hall? If so, I could meet you there. But otherwise, you could just come by my office at 1:30 or I could come to yours when done. Looking forward to seeing all three of you."

- email from SLC colleague, March 1, 2020

Today marks exactly one year since I was last at Sarah Lawrence's campus before the pandemic hit. I've been back there once late in the summer last year, but to pick up some books and materials while clearing out my apartment in Westchester, when the campus was but a ghost town.

March 1, 2020, was also the one and only time that we had brought Matea to the college, so she could meet my colleagues and friends at Sarah Lawrence for the first time. She was only five months back then, still in her infant carrier but already reacting and interacting with total curiosity at everything and everyone. That trip marked a special occasion for us, because it was Matea's first road trip with both of us, and we had driven all the way from Central Illinois to Philadelphia for the Eastern Sociological Association conference, and then continued on from there to Bronxville so I could teach and Matea could get to visit Sarah Lawrence.

That day was so remarkable for us, and me personally, as everything seemed to change since then. It was one of those days where I can remember almost every detail and every conversation, as well as everything that went through my mind. During a lunch with a fellow Malaysian colleague who worked at Sarah Lawrence, we received the news update of a case of COVID-19 near us, a man in New York who lived in nearby Mt. Vernon. At that point in time, it still felt surreal, and we didn't know how to react to such news. We went back to campus to meet a few other colleagues, and I still recall the funny faces and cheerful sounds one of my colleagues made to entertain Matea while a few of us sat and chatted in the common faculty dining room. I remember with great fondness the way Matea would gaze in awe at the tall ceilings in the room from her carrier, and coo adorably at the sight of her own fingers while my colleagues tried to get her attention.

No one mentioned the COVID case that much—it almost didn't seem to register at that point what it all could mean. Certainly not the way things exploded from that point onwards.

Thinking back to a year ago, that first week of March 2020 was also the last time I taught in an actual physical classroom. I had been teaching a once-a-week class on global displacement and refugees, which met Monday evenings for two and half hours in one of the nicer classrooms at Sarah Lawrence's main administration building. I remember that space very well. It would always be dark by the time class began, and we had a large round table and full class of 15, and the students who joined would always come full of energy and enthusiasm. It was a class that taught me that I maybe was mistaken in how I used to think about student participation and engagement levels, that in fact it had a lot to do with the time of day as well—at least at SLC, there are students who actually really enjoy late evening classes, even when they are longer than the usual ninety minutes.

In a way, I am glad that it was my last memory of an actual classroom—a great group of students, a nice space and ambience, and lively conversations driven by genuine interests in the subject topic. A teaching professor's dream. Maybe I'm exaggerating and delusional, thinking wishfully of an idyllic moment that exists mostly in my head…

When we began our drive back to Illinois that week, we had already started receiving updates and rumors about potential lockdowns and quarantine measures, but it was too early to tell what the state of New York was going to do. I remember reacting very badly to Cuomo's "containment" measure at the time, having followed the news out of Wuhan for quite some time and knowing well enough the interconnected character or mobility and movement in New York City. It was like trying to stem a rupture to the carotid with a piece of paper towel.

But I never expected, while driving back across New York, Pennsylvania, Ohio, Indiana and Illinois, that it would be the last time up to now that I'd be seeing the insides of a classroom, the space where I've made my living for so long. That it would be the last time I got to be on that beautiful, quirky college campus for more than a year. As sobering a thought as that is, I'm at a point where it feels much better to look forward to the time I get to take Matea walking in the hilly, uneven but gorgeous college campus and letting her see and play with all the people that make up that community. It will be, as one of my colleagues often puts it, quite the treat.

Parthiban Muniandy

The Panel and the Pandemic

I felt anxious and a bit excited. Instead of the twenty or so attendees I had come to expect at brownbag lunch talks, an audience of more than sixty packed into Weatherhead East Asian Institute's conference room at Columbia University on February 24, 2020. The occasion for this gathering was an interdisciplinary discussion of "the coronavirus epidemic in China and beyond." Tasked by our dispatches collective with returning to an early memory of the pandemic, I am interested in exploring the unease that I initially felt in attending this event. Viewing the recording in 2021 has helped me to connect memories of my personal discomfort to tensions between knowing and doing on the one hand, and individual and collective action on the other.

As the organizer of the event, I had hoped to moderate the discussion, but after one of the invited speakers said she preferred this role, I became a panelist alongside an epidemiologist and public health policy and governance scholar. My jitters on that afternoon were undoubtedly tied to my specific role in the proceeding, and in particular, my qualifications to speak: Whereas my colleagues at the podium in the days leading up to the event had published op-eds in the *New York Times* and collaborated with epidemiologists in Wuhan, I had done little more than casually follow the news and speak with friends who were more directly affected by the early outbreaks.

The opening remarks revealed diverging orientations in the way that we talked about coronavirus. Speaking before me, my co-panelists drew on their disciplinary training to offer fluid and confident commentaries on the spread of the virus in late February 2020. By contrast, my own comments failed to connect the practical questions of the day. The topics I raised—histories of China's responses to SARS and HIV, legacies of Maoist modes of mobilizing citizens, and a troubling past links between infectious disease transmission and with anti-Asian racism—were not unimportant. However, perhaps in part due to an academic habitus honed by years of carefully crafting an ethnographic present for events occurring nearly a decade earlier, I felt ill-equipped and unwilling to translate long-standing disciplinary concerns into recommendations for action.

After our initial introductory remarks, the moderator opened the discussion portion of the event with a two-pronged question that seemed to capture the interests of many in the room. She wondered, first, what "we" should "be looking for in the next few weeks or months," and then asked my co-panelists what she "as a regular person" should be doing in finding a "sensible approach" to living in this moment.

The responses were instructive. The epidemiologist discussed death rates, modes of transmission, population susceptibility, and the possibilities for developing a vaccine. She also outlined potential future prevention measures, including social distancing—a less than familiar term for many at the time—at home and in schools. While in the moment I had found her remarks to be sobering, upon viewing a year later, I was surprised at how much the scientific community already knew about COVID-19 at this point, a week before the first case was confirmed in New York City.

The global health scholar's response highlighted a different set of challenges. Taking up our moderator's question about the future, he provided a comparison between the COVID-19 outbreak and the global reach of SARS. Citing a similar number of countries reporting infections and shared absence of "sustainable community transmission," he concluded that the coronavirus was not yet a global pandemic. SARS, he pointed out, had fizzled out after reaching a similar stage of transmission. Even as the political scientist's analysis carefully built on available data, his SARS comparison for me in 2021 evoked the exceptionalism that so many North Americans felt at the time: Whether due to population density, public health resources, cultural traits, voluntarist ethos, or superior medical technology, we might be saved from the virus.

At the time, I remember being struck by how sharply this assessment contrasted with other ways of intuiting the future. In particular, I thought of recent conversations with a friend who had recently relocated to Vancouver. Obsessively following the news cycle back at home in China, he was increasingly alarmed by the laissez-faire response of local governments and told me with a visceral certainty that North America would suffer enormously.

The panel ended with a wishful question from an audience member about seasonality of the virus (could summer save us?) and an ominous reference to the growing role of rumor in influencing broader understandings of the virus. Another audience member asked a question about the prospects of organizing a global summit of senior leaders to coordinate prevention and treatment efforts. Listening a year later, I found this suggestion of building a comprehensive global response to the pandemic to be at once poignant and infuriating in light of the subsequent failures to coordinate on anything from travel regulations to vaccine distribution.

After the event, lines of people hoping to ask more questions formed in front of the other panelists. The only person who approached me was an older man. Unhappy with the direction of our discussion, he questioned my decision to organize a panel that didn't explicitly focus on highlighting the work of humanitarian organizations. The event might have helped raise money for others in need. "Why do you organize a meeting just to talk? Something needs to be done!"

This audience member's comment seemed to crystallize a broader set of shared anxieties and frustrations in the room. While my presentation had conspicuously failed to speak to our immediate future, the careful and informed responses of my co-panelists also fell short of the group's hunger for actionable knowledge. As "responsible" citizens, those present wanted to participate in a broader "sensible" response. The discomfort that I and others felt on that afternoon came at least in part from confronting increasingly ominous signs about the future of the virus while facing the prospect that a coordinated, collective response would not be materializing.

Nicholas Bartlett

Blue Fade, Fragments

March 1, 2020

Hello from Copenhagen! Everything went smoothly with the flight, and arriving at the apartment. I like the flat a lot—it's comfortable and quiet, and in an interesting neighborhood. It's good to be here, even with the typical jetlag disorientation. I hope to get a good sleep tonight, and then tomorrow I'll be going to the university. Perhaps soon I'll start feeling eager to get back to writing again.

- from a WhatsApp message to a friend, far away

March 1, 2021

"Effective Monday, March 16th, this Bow Tie Cinema will be closed."

The sign caught my eye as I was walking past the entrance to the cinema in the village center close to where I now live, in New York. The glass doors are shut fast, the ticket booth empty. At first, I thought the closing date was for this current month. But I later realized that the notice was from March 2020—the 16th was on a Monday that year. The theatre has apparently remained closed since then. Large glossy posters are still up, advertisements from the films that were circulating or "coming soon" in those days, set in glass frames along the facades of the building. I do not recognize the titles. "Free Guy." "Onward." "The French Dispatch." The movie posters carry the tonalities of a fading blue, a pale, off-tint aqua from late day radiance, a year's worth of photonic erosion, ongoing.

March 6, 2020

I've been spending a lot of time on my own, which is starting to get to me. Moods of feeling kind of down, mixed with moments of feeling excited to be here.

I just saw it. Oh no. What are your thoughts on it?

"COVID is weird," said a friend recently, or just the other day. The virus shifts, alters, moves and affects in quirky, spiky, cryptic ways. The virus sneaks up on people, hits them hard, returns with renewed force, or barely glances upon them. The pandemic has wracked havoc in people's lives; the pandemic sickens, and sickens further; or it haunts the quiet edges of existence; its viral potential lingers like a specter, a phantasmal glimmer of illness, death, impairment, transformation. The virus has the potential to mutate wildly, dangerously; some variants are now spreading across a global expanse.

"COVID doesn't care." Or so says a medical scholar, knowledgeable of its unsentimental ways, in stressing that the virus cares not the slightest for the concerns or strivings of human beings in responding to ravages in their suddenly shaky lifeworlds.

- the first two paragraphs of an afterword I am writing, for a collection of anthropological essays on "transformative experience"

March 9, 2020

And then earlier this evening I spoke with my friend A., by Skype. Which was good. She's from Milan, and she's worried about the situation there. Her parents are there.

Yes, I saw [the reports on Italy closing down]. That happened just after we said goodbye—as she hadn't heard of it.

It's a strange time.

I saw one video, with the women fighting [in a store, over seemingly scarce rolls of toilet paper].

Maybe in a way I'm on a deserted island now, while in Copenhagen, isolated, but serene.

March 10, 2021

She is the last one I would have expected to have died, young, and—this could be—of her own choosing. She always appeared to be happy, and would greet me with a bright smile whenever I saw her.

I cannot say that I knew her well. There was a quietness to her.

March 12, 2020

"Trump's announcement?" Wow. I just saw the headline [on President Trump's announcement on restrictions on travel from Europe].

The US ban on travel from Europe applies "only to foreigners"??!

Somehow, I imagine that when I step outside, it will be like the day after the zombie apocalypse—no one on the streets, an eerie wind blowing through empty fields...

March 13, 2020

The university here has closed down for the next couple of weeks, at least, with courses switching to virtual formats. This doesn't affect me too much, but it does mean that I can't work from my office there, or participate in any events or gatherings. So mostly now I am working at home—wondering if the virus is silently circulating about…

Internal exile now. Feeling okay. Kind of isolated, and a bit bored, but okay. Trying to employ "social distancing" techniques; wondering if I should stop going to cafes (but then that would mean more isolation...)

How are you?

It's unclear to me how she died. There has been no direct word on that.

March 15, 2020

I'm working at home this morning. (thinking that being in crowded cafes is not such a good idea any longer ...)

But it looks like people are now becoming very cautious, and minimizing interactions, keeping a safe distance. (In the market today I noticed a man, with his coat hood on, in the checkout line, standing a good two meters away from the person in front of him—he then bought a pack of cigarettes...)

March 16

Yes. I was thinking this morning that if this was a movie, there would be a sign saying something like "Day 5" (and counting...)

What will "Day 42" be like...?

We are at Day 371 now, and counting…

March 17, 2020

Hey. I'm ok, I guess. Making do with this new world not ours. Trying to not feel too isolated. (I've gone to work at cafes yesterday afternoon, and today, which helps, despite the possible risks of that). How are you?

Yeah, something like that. Communal isolation. I find that my brain starts fading into the white walls if and when I spend too much time at home with just my own thoughts and faint presence in play. But it does help knowing that others throughout the world are facing much the same.

I do find that my mood is better if I can work at a cafe for a couple hours each day (or something like that), compared to being and working at home all day. Then, I start feeling gloomy, sad, and dis-attentive. Like a monkey kept in a cage, with no companions around, and nothing engaging to do....

The lyrics and melody of Elton John's song, "Someone saved my life tonight," have been circling through my mind.

March 18, 2020

Everything is more in a lock-down here, starting this morning. "All cafes must remain closed." Sigh.

"Have you heard from T. today? He's been calling everyone. I think he's lonely."
"That's his fault."
- an exchange overheard, this afternoon

March 20, 2020

The first real in-person conversation for me in two weeks.

It's kind of them to invite me. I think the word is out that I'm alone here, and would welcome company now and then.

"It's after the second vaccination shot that some people feel somewhat sick, afterwards. That's what people say. That was the case for me. I felt a bit feverish a few hours later, with aches and pains—malaise, you know. And then after a day and half it went away, so that was good."

March 23, 2020

How have you been sleeping? Yes, I find it all very tiring, especially when I read the news reports, which I do several times a day—waves upon waves of hardship, illness, anxiety, and uncertainty. When I'm asleep I'm oblivious to it all, but then upon waking this morning I felt "queasy," a bit nauseous—a limit or stoppage of "breath," perhaps, as you've noted. Such strangeness, yes, in this Copenhagen, quiet streets, people walking mutely about, looking stunned.

Through all this I am very appreciative of the fact that you and I can stay in touch, and be in touch, through words. It's a lifeline of sorts, which keeps me afloat.

The idea for a book, morbidly, incandescent, 'the anthropology of my suicide.' What such a work might entail is terribly intriguing, and frightening.
Leave it.

March 23, 2020

Good question. Soon, I hope. Maybe late May or early June is a time that we can "within reason" think it's possible, once the world settles down again? What do you think?

It's true but it's difficult to know at all what the world will be like through the summer months. But I think that in a few weeks' time they will become clearer, as to whether things are getting better, or worse, or just continued restrictions.

...Everything seemed so carefree, then—

I can relate better to what people went through during World War II—not seeing family and loved ones for months, or years, worrying about their welfare, from afar.

March 24

So far, so good. Quiet, solitudinal, as usual these days.

all media saddens me

March 25, 2020

Yes, it's overwhelming [in New York City]. They're being hit very hard there. My friend A. is there, and she has not left her apartment (in Harlem) in some 10 days now. Playing it safe.

March 26, 2020

I find something similar these days with writing. It's a space and time for calm focus, imaginative rendering, intellectual challenge. And with this I can forget the current state of emergency in the world, for an hour or two at a time.

Yes, now that you mention it. My words, and the words of others, are good company. Sometimes undisciplined, and unruly, but they are there, in a good way. Survivance, yes.

Right. And in a strange, unexpected way, the crisis has offered me something I was looking for, at this time. A quiet space to think, write, reflect, and write some more.

You shouldn't worry about me. I'm doing okay. I don't feel sad, or "down." I'm a bit surprised by that, but it's true. And it's been really good to visit some friends lately.

March 27, 2021

"Suicide and Self-Harm: Bereaved Families Count the Costs of Lockdowns." The psychological toll on young people of months in isolation and great global suffering is becoming clearer after successive lockdowns.

"A 19-year-old history student at Cardiff University, Lily was self-confident, outgoing and charismatic in public, her friends and family said, but as she went back to school in September, she began to struggle with the effects of lockdown…."

"'Lockdown put Lily in physical and emotional situations she would never have in normal times,' said Lily's mother, Annie."[3]

March 28

"B.1.1.7 is really scary."

March 29

Disaster medicine.

March 30, 2020

Things are getting more locked down. They've been talking about the "two-person" limit here, as well, but they haven't implemented it.

I'm doing okay. A cross-section of my mind might reveal various regions of subdued, engaged, bored, aloneness, distant sociality, anxious concern (mostly for others), hope for a better situation soon, fears of getting sick (myself), longing, anticipation, desire, searching for creativity...

The pandemic has changed people's lives, often through events and processes of "radical rupture." Some persons and families have been rendered financially broke, or existentially broken; others have found new arrangements in life and relations to others. Plans and life projects—work, study, travel, family—have been cancelled, delayed; deferred, rerouted, revamped. Rites of transition—graduation ceremonies, weddings, of birth, death, aging—have been altered, refashioned. The pandemic has thrown into sharp relief inequalities of income, class, job and food security, and access to health care. With all this comes inquietude; moments of despair, and scenes of resiliency, creative making and renewal; exhaustion, weariness, separation, isolation; new arrange-

ments of space and time; new connections and forms of communication, virtual or viral. People have been estranged from the lives that they would want to live, if they could do so. Many are living in exile from the lives they once knew and took as self-evident. Some are stuck in particular circuits of time, or find themselves mired in limited, confined spaces and reduced to repetitive quadrants of action and non-action. Through the pandemic, experience has been rendered weird, as has the idea and phenomena of transformative experiences.

- The third paragraph of the afterword on transformative experience[4]

March 31, 2020

Yes, I'm going to write for a few hours now. On "phantasms," for one. It's coming along, slowly. Just need to keep working at it. It looks like I'll be on my own through this week, but maybe I'll see some folks on the weekend.

"The New Normal in N.Y.: High Virus Rates and a Steady Stream of Cases. As New York races to vaccinate residents while variants spread, the state's positive test rate and case counts are likely to remain stable for a while."

It's bad in NYC right now. My friends and colleagues appear to be doing okay, so far. Everyone is "sheltering in place," and my colleagues are teaching remotely. All is good with my family in Massachusetts. I'll call my mother later today, to say hello. Thanks for asking.

"COVID IS STILL HERE"

-words flashing on an electronic billboard set along the Westside Highway in New York City

Robert Desjarlais

A Different Kind of Red

February 20, 2021

I walk briskly along the Martesana canal with my dog on the leash, through the damp and chill of the evening. The weather is strange these days, an anticyclone conjures the illusion of a premature spring, but at dusk the warmer temperatures drop, restoring a sense of the Milanese winter, which always feels much colder than its actual temperature, whether you measure it in Celsius or Fahrenheit.

As usual, during my dog walks, my brain is set on a wakeful alertness mode. My state of consciousness blends with Baldo's as we both stay on vigilant guard, in anticipation of an imminent event: a skirmish with another quadruped, the sight (and the possible chase) of a muskrat, the detection of another dog's "calling card" and the sudden fascination with the new smell. Although this rich array of canine stimuli translates for me into the far less enjoyable experience of a sudden and vigorous pull of the leash, I need to stay focused and be prepared to the physical effort that a dog fight or a hunting chase generally entail.

Sometimes during these walks, I forget about the more complex layers of my extended consciousness of the past and the future and I just focus on *the feeling of what happens*.[5] Other times, like tonight, something disrupts my unelaborated dog-walk consciousness: I detect something that does not belong to the canine semiotic landscape. *What is this?* I wonder to myself as I gaze at the familiar-yet-unidentified object. As I re-emerge from my mimetic dive into Baldo's consciousness, I momentarily struggle to find the name and meaning of the colorful fragments of paper scattered on the sidewalk… *Confetti! That's what they are!* I contemplate the traces of a fugacious and inconspicuous children's parade. This year's carnival has gone by and I haven't even realized it. Carnival… I actually forgot such a thing existed.

February 20, 2020

It's Shrove Tuesday—in most regions of Italy, that's Carnival. Streets are filled with little flocks of masqueraded kids proudly parading their costumes. I never liked carnivals when I was little. "Il Coronavirus è arrivato in Lombardia," says a stranger's familiar voice as I wake up to the sound of the Italian radio I like to listen to (in streaming) from my Harlem apartment. Since I returned to New York City in early January, I have been hearing reports about a mysterious atypical form of pneumonia spreading in China. Now *it has arrived in Lombardy*, the region where most of my family and friends live. Trains no longer stop at the stations of Codogno and Casalpusterlengo—where the first cluster outbreaks have been identified. My two biggest fears have materialized. The precarious quality of my transnational affective existence is now fully exposed to the specters of planetary disease and boundaries shutdown.

February 27, 2020

A day of almost uninterrupted teaching is turning to an end. I am in my office waiting for R. to come and pick me up. Our schedules are always packed with classes and individual meetings with students and we rarely get to meet on campus, without making proper arrangements. I always look forward to our evening get-togethers and to the comfort of a spirited chat and a cold Sapporo with my good colleague and friend. But tonight there is a different kind of intensity surrounding our meeting. I am waiting for R. with greater excitement, not only because he will soon take off to spend his sabbatical in Denmark, but also because I am getting worried about the spread of the contagion in Europe.

Earlier in the day during a meeting of the Diversity Committee of which I am a member I felt particularly disconnected, as if I were in a different affective bubble from that of my American interlocutors. They were still operating as if the virus was far away. But I was charged with a different intensity—one that stemmed from attachments and my exposure to the news coming from Europe's viral epicenter.

February 27, 2021

The evening at Wild Ginger with R. was pleasant as usual, but became memorable in retrospect: a last supper in ways that I could never foresee at the time, the last convivial encounter I had before the unraveling of my social world.

March 1, 2020

Please be careful when you go out, Aurora, Coronavirus has arrived in NYC. I receive a text from my friend Lili. As I imagined, it did not take long for this news to arrive. I pause to think about the current dissemination of an anthropocentric narrative of viral contagion—one that gives anthropomorphic qualities to a non-human and non-living entity. No one knows when the virus actually began to spread in the city. But our media-driven chronology merges the date of the first confirmed case with the alleged date of the virus arrival.[6] Somewhat amused, I imagine the virus at a JFK carousel picking up his luggage and heading toward the exit.

I look back at my phone screen with a strange mixture of fear and relief. I shiver as I think of the city's human density, the subway, the weekend lines at Trader Joe's; at the same time, I find myself hoping that this fictitious scene of viral arrival will end the solitude originating from my inhabiting the proximate future of the Italian mediascape.

March 16, 2020

News from a different timespace: a video about the virus is becoming viral. "It is believed that the U.S., England, and France are 9 to 10 days behind Italy in COVID-19 progression," reads the video's opening statement in English. The footage shows an assemblage of short clips by quarantined Italians speaking to their selves of 10 days ago.[7] The English subtitles suggest, however, an ecumenical audience: *Hi Daniele-from-10-days-ago … I am speaking to you from the future… A huge mess is about to happen… I am sure you already heard of Coronavirus and I am also pretty sure you are underestimating it. Hospitals are blowing up… I know China is far away, but the virus is faster than what you think…* The words give shape to a new world of slightly differed synchronicity.

March 26, 2021

There has been a total shift in Italian public moral discourse. Twelve months ago, a wave of public indignation would target those who, in open violation of the lockdown measures, were caught jogging or exercising outdoors.[8] Now the stigma is on those who are cowardly compliant with the restrictive norms. *Are you seeing people? Are you going out? No, I am not. I am not vaccinated yet, though I wish I were.* The invisible enemy is no longer the virus, but the state authority and its abstruse legislative efforts to contain the epidemiological emergency. People are tired and public defiance is explicitly or indirectly glorified. *This is a different kind of red… it not the red of last year's lockdown. People these days tend to think they can go out as they please and do not respect the containment measurements.* We are still mandated to shelter in place, but with a different emphasis and intensity— no longer capable of eliciting a sense of synchronic communality, the restrictive measures are met with boredom, disdain, and anger. Gone are the days when everyone felt part of the same momentous state of emergency. The longest, slowest apocalypse ever imagined—a diluted shade of red.

Aurora Donzelli

Narrating Vaccinations

February 24, 2021

My father called me today from the small town in Northern Italy where he lives. He was enthusiastic to tell me that he received a text message from the health authorities of Treviso, saying that on March 3rd, 2021, he will receive his first dose of the COVID-19 Pfizer vaccine. His intonation and fast speech pace betrayed his happiness. His wife received her first dose today. In Veneto, one of the twenty regions of Italy, they have just started to vaccinate people who were born in 1940–1941. It is their turn now.

This news makes me very happy. I would feel terribly guilty to receive the COVID-19 vaccine before my parents. I am not an essential worker. I have been protecting myself by wearing my masks, by keeping distance from others, and by avoiding too many trips to stores, supermarkets, and other gatherings. Without a vaccine, I really have no choice but to protect myself. Italy is far behind with the distribution of the COVID-19 vaccines. Yet, people who have received this immunization and who will receive it in the next months are lucky and privileged. There are no vaccines in many countries across the world.

"By mid-April, I might be able to have my life back again, at least partially," my father said "I am always in fear, I get tested continuously and I have been staying away from my friends and family. I will at least be more protected with this vaccine!"

I could imagine his satisfied smile on his face. I miss seeing that smile in person. I could feel his emotions through his words as if, for a moment, he could see the end of a tunnel, the arrival after a challenging run, his survival through a pandemic of unimaginable proportions. He will be able to say, "I made it." He will be remembered in the future as one of the old people in Italy who made it. He has just turned 80. Unlike mine this past year, his life has always been very social: he likes to go out for dinner, to be with people, to spend his weekends outside with his friends. He is retired now and his life was very active before the coronavirus hit Italy. He has been stuck in his region for more than a year now. One lockdown after another. The numbers of infections and of deaths have not improved. They are always very high. It has been a tragic reality.

Yet, the fight against COVID-19 won't be over after my father gets his vaccination. It will take some time, perhaps another year. After all, pharmacoepidemiology has made great progress by developing at least six or seven valuable vaccines in less than a year. It usually takes a couple of years to develop a vaccine. There were no vaccines in 1918 when humans were trying to fight the 1918–1920 flu pandemic. They had to resort to cloth masks, to isolation, to being socially distant. The first influenza vaccines were developed many years later, in 1942. Scientific milestones to fight the flu. With COVID-19, scientists are now predicting what is unpredictable. Will we be out of this nightmare in the Summer 2021? Will the COVID-19 pandemic end in September 2021? We still don't know. There are still too many variables, including some very aggressive variants of the virus, that are making our future too volatile. Yet, we might see some light at the end of this interminable tunnel. Knowing that my father has his vaccinal protection will make this light more visible. Being a retired doctor, he has always believed in medicine and science. He was the one who vaccinated my brother and myself when we were kids to protect us from various diseases. He is now among the ones who are thought deserving of protection against the coronavirus and its many variants.

Sabina M. Perrino

The Gray Man Chasing Vaccine Rainbows

The night before the vaccines arrived in Tunis, on March 8th, 2021, the COVID curfew was extended from 8:00 p.m. to 10:00 p.m. It was also the night my friend Noureddine celebrated his 29th birthday with his twin sister, mother, and father. The twins came of age during the 2011 revolution, compelling him to leave his studies in computer science first to study law and then photojournalism. We had met four or five years ago, at that time of the afternoon when people in Tunis avoid being outside. We drank espresso on Monji Slim Street near the church turned boxing gym, and talked leftist politics in Tunisia. I had been struck by his love for his craft. The gray in his hair. And, his chain smoking. Marlboro. Red and ready-rolled.

The sky on March 9th hung low. The day the vaccines had arrived, one month later than expected, Noureddine was with two friends, photojournalists, more experienced and older than he. When we spoke on the phone soon after, he told me that he was dressed, as usual, in his standard blue but operating with light gear, two Fujifilm X-T2 and two lenses. "Why blue?" I asked him. "Do you know the gray man theory? It's about being able to disappear into a crowd but also," he joked, "the life of an introvert." The three of them were photographing a demonstration in front of the Prime Minister's Office in the Kasbah when one of them received a call that the vaccines were arriving mid-afternoon. They had just enough time for lunch before the three friends piled into a Kia Rio and drove to the airport. The police directed them to the tarmac where the photographers and journalists were instructed to stay within a tight perimeter. It was impossible to move around the airfield to shoot. At half-past three, the Minister of Heath received an AirFrance cargo plane with 30,000 doses. Five or six boxes of Sputnik 5. Enough for 15,000 people.

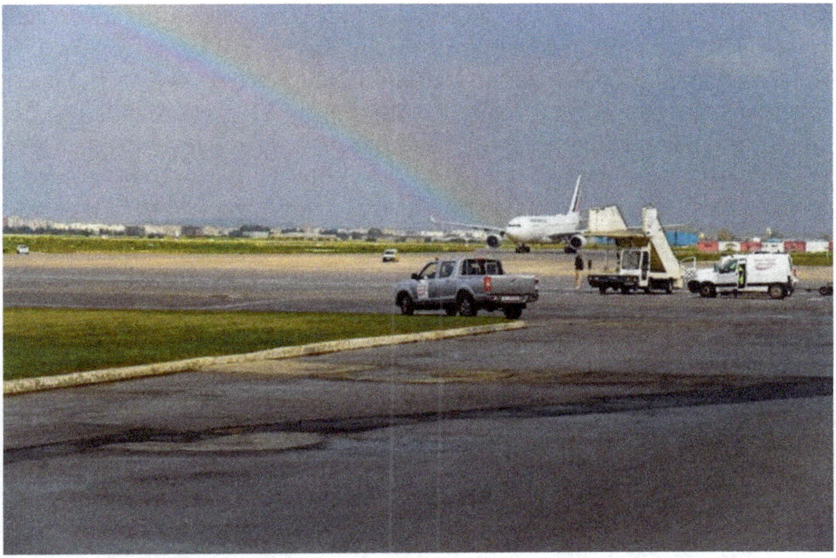

Fig. 5.2 Tunis-Carthage International Airport, March 9, 2021. (Photo by Noureddine Ahmed)

"All this," Noureddine said, "for one little trolly of vaccines, one month-late." Even so, he told me, "I wandered off, looking for THE shot" (Fig. 5.2). The blue-gray man in action.

Margaux Fitoussi

Placing the Javits Center

I am sitting in the last row of chairs in the mandated waiting area minutes after receiving my second shot, taking fieldnotes and reflecting upon two visits to this cavernous space. In my first visit here last month, I had the feeling that this conference-center-turned-mass-vaccination-site functioned as a paradigmatic "non-place." Marc Augé deploys this term to describe transitory spaces that produce in their users the experience of anonymous individuality.[9]

Passing through the Javits center during my first visit evoked a familiar, not entirely unpleasant sense of isolation in a crowd while conjuring associations and uncanny resonances with other mass transitory spaces. The multiple checkpoints, prominent rules and prohibitions, continual surveillance of bodies, and above all the constant starts and stops of navigating the demarcated sections of this reconfigurable space made me feel like a passenger trying to catch a flight. After showing a guard my ID and appointment letter, I joined a line that that snaked back and forth between seemingly endless rows of retractable belt barriers. A man who arrived a few minutes after me was directed into a separate lane free of other visitors. My immediate thought was that he must be a first-class ticket holder, or perhaps he was late and at risk of missing his flight. I realized a minute later that he had elected to get the less popular Johnson and Johnson single shot. No waiting required.

After a half hour of starting and stopping, I reached the check-in area. As I waited, innocuous classical music was periodically punctuated by a calm woman's voice intoning: "We are all in this together. Wear a mask, practice social distancing." More than 200 tables had been arranged in rows, each staffed by a single attendant operating a computer. Employees turned on lamps to signal when they were free to check a new person in. Line coordinators calling out desk numbers in this section made me feel like a weary shopper moving through a Trader Joes check-out line.

Arriving in the area where shots were administered helped me grasp the scale of the operation. One of the 600 New York National Guard members working at the site barked at me to hurry to Station 8—I instinctively broke into a jog. An exhausted nurse greeted me by saying, "you are too soon!" and gestured for me to move back as she sprayed a chair with a disinfectant. She then turned to a colleague, declared, "I'm done!" and walked away. Another nurse quickly came over to take her place, and within less than five minutes I had my shot and vaccination card in hand and was being ushered into the post-shot waiting area and then back onto the street. If anthropological notions of place were premised on organic connection that built relational identity, the notion of "non-place" captured my experience as a member of an anonymous crowed moving toward a shared destination in a state of "solitary contractuality."[10]

My second visit three weeks later leads me to revisit my initial characterization of this space. The shift started with me. Back in April, weeks removed from constantly refreshing my browser in attempt to secure evanescent appointment times, I had rushed to 42nd street to ensure I arrived on time. This initial visit occurred just forty eight hours before the country would hit its all-time high of 3.38 million people vaccinated in a single day in a national campaign desperate to meet demand for shots. By contrast, now nearly two weeks into May, I am aware that local governments are moving to "downscale" mega-vaccination sites. In efforts to actively seek out unvaccinated populations, mobile clinics are moving into a range of neighborhood settings. I have recurring thought that, as a partially vaccinated citizen, the government needs me to reach their own targets as much as I need them. Unhurried in my morning routines, I arrive at the center two hours after my appointment time.

On this visit, I am acutely aware of how the movement of people in the vast hall is shaped by connections to the outside world. Upon arriving, signs at the entrance announce that there are hundreds of walk-in spots available today. The crowd has greatly diminished; I learn that the center today will vaccinate 4,000 people less than on my last visit. A reconfigured floor plan now allows me to walk in straight, short bursts between sections. Most of what I described above—the music and announcements, the stations, and procedures—was unchanged. But people appear to inhabit the spaces differently. Workers are relaxed, even distracted. A registration employee is engrossed in her Danielle Steele novel, a woman seated at the translator booth is doing her homework. Members of the National Guard crack jokes with each other rather than offering visitors stern lectures about putting away phones. With no one yelling instructions at us, visitors moving towards our vaccines also seem much more at ease.

Within fifteen minutes of my arrival at the center, I receive my second shot and enter the post-vaccination waiting area. Other visitors sit silently, many stare into the glow of screens. Craving connection while consigned to my seat, I wonder how others in this waiting area might be feeling about their visit. I suddenly think of TurboVax—the computer programmer and Twitter hero who helped tens of thousands of New Yorkers find shots. In his twitter feed, he described the Javits center as the "Real Vaccine Experience" and insisted on receiving his two doses here. The "non-place" aspects of the Javitz Center allowing it to deliver more jabs than any other center in the country for him are a testimony to the uniqueness of this centrally located convention center and the achievements of New York City's historic response. I find I am suddenly feeling a sense of affection for this space and the people who are briefly passing through.

I have lingered in the waiting area for nearly an hour. A newly vaccinated group will soon fill up the seats around me. I move slowly to the exit, suddenly sad to say goodbye to an operation I know will soon be gone.

Nicholas Bartlett

Notes

1. Rabinow (1996).
2. Caillois (1966).
3. https://www.nytimes.com/2021/03/27/world/europe/suicide-self-harm-pandemic.html?searchResultPosition=4
4. Desjarlais (2021).
5. Damasio (1999).
6. Goldstein J. and McKinley J. "Coronavirus in N.Y.: Manhattan Woman Is First Confirmed Case in State", New York Times, March 1, 2020. https://www.nytimes.com/2020/03/01/nyregion/new-york-coronvirus-confirmed.html? (last accessed, April 3, 2022).
7. https://www.youtube.com/watch?v=o_cImRzKXOs (last accessed, April 3, 2022).
8. One of the most emblematic cases concerned the footage of a man exercising outdoors on deserted beach aired lived during an afternoon show. The TV host publicly condemned the jogger who was being chased by a police helicopter. https://www.huffingtonpost.it/entry/linseguimento-in-diretta-su-pomeriggio-5-scatena-lira-dei-social_it_5e957564c5b60e5553ab5000 (last accessed, April 3, 2022).
9. Augé (1995).
10. Augé (1995: 94).

Postscript

It

For nearly the entirety of 2021, I could not write for this project. Glancing at the collective manuscript now, I see that the last time I wrote was four days after the storming of the Capitol, which would have been the tenth of January. It is now the end of December. Round after round of our textual exchanges, I found myself passing my turn. What was there left to say? The virus is still surging. The virus is waning. We have defeated the virus. We have been defeated. Some have died. Some have lived. Military personnel at mass vaccination centers. Another sprawling "tent city." Delta, and now Omicron, skipping two letters in between, it is rumored, to avert the fatal movement of the alphabet, and its beeline for potential offense to the Xi administration.

Perhaps the paralysis struck after a particular genre of violence, newly circulating imagistically—the shoving of Asian American elders into the pavement, at times to their death—would not leave my mind. The first few cases to reach the news hit in northern California. A man in his 80s, of Thai descent, knocked to the ground near his home in San Francisco, leading to brain hemorrhaging and death several days later. A man in his 90s in Oakland Chinatown, thrust in the same manner into the sidewalk. A man in his 70s, of Chinese descent, pushed to the pavement in Oakland's Lake Merritt on his morning stroll, to his death. Shove after shove cropped up on my digital feed in the days and months that followed, adding to the

R. Desjarlais et al., *Dispatches from Home and the Field during the COVID-19 Pandemic*, Palgrave Studies in Literary Anthropology,
https://doi.org/10.1007/978-3-031-19193-0

other forms of violence already populating it. As the prompts to write for this volume rotated to me, no words came. Or rather, words were superfluous. They rang superficial, clanging of a sound somewhere between metal and plastic, dropping off of anything they touched.

In "Why I Write," Joan Didion says this of the title she "stole" from George Orwell:[1]

I like the sound of the words… There you have three short unambiguous words that share a sound, and the sound they share is this:

I

I

I

Writing, she continues, is an aggressive act—an imposition of the *I*, no matter its turns of stylistic evasion. But soon, another tyrant enters the scene. Grammar, she tells us, holds infinite power, inflexibly altering what is said and meant through its arrangements. Then again, grammar reveals itself to be mere instrument to another despotic force: the picture. "The picture dictates the arrangements":

> It tells you.
>
> You don't tell it.

The picture dictates what is to be found through the shape of a sentence—whether it "ends hard" or with a "dying-fall." In my case, with one picture of a dying-fall after the next, flashing in their dictation, the writing ended hard. Now, nearly a year later, the *I* finds itself stepping on the stones of grammar again. But to say what?

There could be many things to say. And many things have been well said by others across mediums. But like other nagging hollows since the start of COVID times, and since far before, some things fall and fall into them more so than they come up for air. An *I* finds the act of imposition impossible in the face of an *It*, and even grammar sits still, withdrawing its arrangements.

Emily Ng
December 2021

Note

1. Didion, Joan. 1976. "Why I Write." *The New York Times,* December 5, 1976 (https://www.nytimes.com/1976/12/05/archives/why-i-write-why-i-write.html).

References

Appadurai, Arjun. 2013. *The Future as Cultural Fact: Essays on the Global Condition*. New York: Verso.

Augé, Marc. 1995. *Non-Places: Introduction to an Anthropology of Supermodernity*. Translated by John Howe. New York: Verso Press.

Barthes, Roland. 1994. *Roland Barthes by Roland Barthes*. Trans. Richard Howard. Berkeley: University of California Press.

Benjamin, Walter. 1999. *The Arcades Project*. Trans. Howard Eiland & Kevin McLaughlin, Cambridge, MA. & London: Belknap Press.

———. 2016. *One-Way Street*. Cambridge: Belknap Press.

Bourgois, Philippe and Jeff Schonberg. 2009. *Righteous Dopefiend*. Berkeley, Los Angeles and London: University of California Press.

Cabral, Amilcar. 1973. *Return to the Source*. New York: Monthly Review Press.

Caillois, Roger. 1966. *Pierres*. Paris: Gallimard.

Camus, Albert. 1947. *La Peste*. Paris, France: Gallimard.

Carlson, Jen. 2020. Video: How Brooklyn's Biggest 7 O'Clock 'Covid-Release Block Party Began. *Gothamist,* 2 July 2020, Gothamist.com/arts-entertainment/video-how-brooklyns-biggest-7-oclock-covid-release-block-party-began.

Damasio, Antonio. 1999. *The Feeling of What Happens*. New York: Harcourt.

Davis, Wade. 2020. The Unraveling of America. *Rolling Stone*, August 6, 2020.

Deaglio, Enrico. 2019. *La Bomba*: Cinquant'anni di Piazza Fontana. Milano: Feltrinelli Editore.

Dean, Jodi. 2019. *Comrade*. New York: Verso.

Derrida, Jacques. 1981. *Disseminations*. Chicago: University of Chicago Press.

R. Desjarlais et al., *Dispatches from Home and the Field during the COVID-19 Pandemic*, Palgrave Studies in Literary Anthropology, https://doi.org/10.1007/978-3-031-19193-0

Desjarlais, Robert. 2011. *Counterplay*: An Anthropologist at the Chessboard. Berkeley: University of California Press.

Desjarlais, Robert. 2021. The years of living transformatively. *Ethos* 49: 368–376.

Didion, Joan. 1976. Why I Write. *The New York Times*, December 5, 1976.

Durkheim, Émile. 1995 [1912]. *The Elementary Forms of Religious Life*. The Free Press: New York.

Fraser, Gordon. 2020. Conspiracy, pornography, democracy: the recurrent aesthetics of the American Illuminati. *Journal of American Studies* 54 (2): 273–294.

Freud, Sigmund. 1955. Notes upon a case of obsessional neurosis. In *The Standard Edition of the Complete Psychological Works of Sigmund Freud, Volume X (1909): Two Case Histories ('Little Hans' and the 'Rat Man')*, 151–318.

Gordillo, Gaston. 2014. *Rubble: The Afterlife of Destruction*. Durham: Duke University Press.

Gottleib, Alma. 1995. Beyond the Lonely Anthropologist: Collaboration in Research and Writing. *American Anthropologist* 97 (1): 21–26.

Herr, Michael. 1977. *Dispatches*. New York: Knopf.

Hofstadter, Richard. 1964. The paranoid style in American politics. *Harper's Magazine*, November 36

Jacomé, Jorge, and Garbiñe Ortega. 2020. Jorge Jácome 'Fiesta Forever." *Interview*, V-Drome, 18 June 2020. www.vdrome.org/jorge-jacome.

Kaplan, Martha. 2007. Fijian water in Fiji and New York: Local politics and a global commodity. *Cultural Anthropology* 22 (4): 685–706.

Klima, Alan. 2002. *The Funeral Casino: Meditation, Massacre, and Exchange with the Dead in Thailand*. Princeton: Princeton University Press.

Lareau, Annette. 2011. *Unequal Childhoods: Class, Race and Family Life, with an update a decade later*. University of California Press.

Lévi-Strauss, Claude. 1963. The Effectiveness of Symbols. In *Structural anthropology*. Trans. Clair Jacobson and Brooke Grundfest Schope. New York: Basic Books.

Luc, Jean-Nancy. 2002. *Being Singular Plural*. Stanford University Press.

Mosna-Savoye, Géraldine. 2020. J'ai eu la nostalgie de la fête. *Carnet De Philo, France Culture*, 2 October 2020. www.franceculture.fr/emissions/carnet-de-phio/la-chronique-philo-du-vendredi-02-octobre-2020.

Moten, Fred. 2017. *Black and Blur (consent not to be a single being)*. Durham: Duke University Press.

Povinelli, Elizabeth A. 2006. *The empire of love: Toward a theory of intimacy, genealogy, and carnality*. NC: Duke University Press.

Rabinow, Paul. 1996. *Essays on the Anthropology of Reason*. Princeton: Princeton University Press.

Rosner, Elizabeth. 2020. Hundreds Gather for Secret Rave under NYC's Kosciuszko Bridge. *New York Post*, 3 August 2020. nypost.com/2020/08/03/hundreds-gather-for-secret-rave-under-nycs-kosciuszko-bridge.

Sedgwick, Eve Kosofsky. 2003. *Touching feeling*. Duke University Press.
Stewart, Kathleen. 2008. *Ordinary Affects*. Durham: Duke University Press.
Vico, Giambattista. 1725. *Principj di una Scienza Nuova Intorno alla Natura delle Nazioni*. Naples: Felice Mosca.
Wong, Michael, Vishi Gnanakumaran, and Daniel Goldreich. 2011. Tactile Spatial Acuity Enhancement in Blindness: Evidence for Experience-Dependent Mechanisms. *Journal of Neuroscience* 31 (19): 7028–7037. https://doi.org/10.1523/JNEUROSCI.6461-10.2011.
Yurchak, Alexei. 2005. *Everything Was Forever, Until It Was No More: The Last Soviet Generation*. Princeton: Princeton University Press.

CPSIA information can be obtained
at www.ICGtesting.com
Printed in the USA
LVHW081632030223
738603LV00006B/551

9 783031 191923